NUTRITION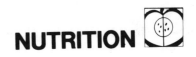

Other Preventive Medicine Institute/Strang Clinic
HEALTH ACTION PLANS

 How to Stop Smoking

Personal and Family Safety and Crime Prevention

Physical Fitness

NUTRITION

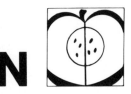

A Preventive Medicine Institute/Strang Clinic
HEALTH ACTION PLAN

CHERYL CORBIN, M.S., R.D.
Director of Nutrition
PMI/Strang Clinic

Series Editor
Daniel G. Miller, M.D.

Associate Editors
Marilyn Snyder Halper, M.P.H.
Pamela Hatch
Ira Neiger

Holt, Rinehart and Winston   New York

First published in January 1981 by Holt, Rinehart and Winston,
383 Madison Avenue, New York, New York 10017.

Published simultaneously in Canada by Holt, Rinehart and
Winston of Canada, Limited.

Library of Congress Cataloging in Publication Data

Corbin, Cheryl.
   Nutrition.

   (A Preventive Medicine Institute/Strang Clinic
health action plan)
   Bibliography: p.
   Includes index.
   1. Nutrition   I. Title.   II. Series: Preventive
Medicine Institute/Strang Clinic. Preventive Medicine
Institute/Strang Clinic health action plan.
QP141.C748   613.2   80-11138

ISBN Hardbound: 0-03-048281-X
ISBN Paperback: 0-03-048276-3

First Edition

Designer: Betty Binns Graphics
Printed in the United States of America
10 9 8 7 6 5 4 3 2 1

Contents

After more than four years of research, study, and testing, it is with great pride and pleasure that we bring you this Preventive Medicine Institute/Strang Clinic Health Action Plan. The development of this book (one of four currently available) has been one of the most exciting—and, we believe, successful—projects the clinic has ever undertaken. By making use of the Health Action Plans, you will be taking a major step toward improving your own health as well as that of your family.

Taken together, these plans address the health problems—cancer, heart disease, and accidents—responsible for the majority of chronic illnesses, disabilities, and premature deaths in this country. The four books—*Personal and Family Safety and Crime Prevention, How to Stop Smoking, Nutrition,* and *Physical Fitness*—deal directly with the behaviors most closely associated with these health concerns.

Until recently, it has been generally assumed that advanced technology, more physicians, and better medical care would ensure the health and increase the life spans of most Americans. While we have made tremendous progress in the fields of disease detection and cure, and life expectancy has increased dramatically since the turn of the century, considerable evidence indicates that we have reached a point of diminishing returns. Life expectancy has leveled off in the last few decades, and disease patterns have changed. Infectious diseases such as tuberculosis, pneumonia, and typhoid, once among the most feared health problems, have, for the most part, been replaced by chronic disorders such as cancer and heart disease.

The path to the control of chronic diseases lies in a new direction. While we don't have all the answers, we do have hard evidence that links cancer to smoking, implicates high-fat diets and obesity in cancer and heart disease, and suggests that lack of regular exercise contributes to heart and respiratory problems.

To put it another way, the major causes of chronic disease, disability, and death in the Western world have one important thing in common: they are all connected to some extent to our behavior, our habits. Improved health, therefore, unquestionably will depend upon our ability to throw away our cigarettes, change our dietary habits, exercise regularly, and learn to take precautions against avoidable accidents. In today's world, health depends more on our ability to *prevent* diseases and accidents than on our ability to treat their effects once they have occurred. And since the decision to live wisely is an individual's choice, your health, to a great extent, is in your own hands.

Our belief in the concept of preventive medicine led us to develop the Health Action Plans. Many reputable books on related subjects are available, but we believe ours are unique for three reasons. First, their ultimate objective is *permanent* change in everyday health habits and life-styles. Second, each Health Action Plan provides a *structured* approach to behavioral change—a simple, step-by-step way to achieve personal health-related goals. Third, the structure is similar in each of the Health Action Plans, so if you use one, you will find the format of the others familiar, allowing you to readily develop your own *individualized and integrated* programs.

Each book includes a section on self-assessment to give you a deeper understanding of your current habits. Once you have been made aware of the details of these habits, you are given suggestions for making health-improving changes as well as the tools for achieving your specific goals. In addition, each book makes provision for maintaining change once it has been achieved. The maintenance plans often involve record keeping, which not only increases your awareness and knowledge of a health habit, but arms you with additional reinforcement for further change.

All the Health Action Plans were developed with the help of consultants and consumers. People like you were asked to test each plan and to make suggestions. These consumers were discriminating critics, and their contributions benefited the plans greatly. Health consultants—doctors, nutritionists, exercise physiologists, and other experts—have also carefully considered each program, commenting on content and accuracy and helping in program testing.

None of these plans provides an instant answer: rather, they are personally focused programs for modifying the way you live so that you and your family can enjoy long, happy—and healthy lives.

A person's health must ultimately be his or her own responsibility. We hope that these Health Action Plans will provide you with a practical and reliable guide to a healthier life.

Daniel G. Miller, M.D.
Director, Preventive Medicine
Institute/Strang Clinic

A word about the Preventive Medicine Institute/Strang Clinic

The Preventive Medicine Institute/Strang Clinic is a nonprofit organization dedicated to the prevention of cancer, heart disease, stroke, and other serious illnesses. Established at Memorial Hospital in New York City in 1940 by Dr. Elise Strang L'Esperance, the Strang Clinic originally became well known for its pioneering use of the Pap test, the screening technique for cervical cancer devised by Dr. George Papanicolaou. In 1963 the clinic became an independent center. At that time the clinic—which until then had been devoted largely to cancer detection—broadened its scope to cover diagnosis, research, and detection of all the major chronic and controllable diseases. In 1966 the clinic was renamed the Preventive Medicine Institute/Strang Clinic, with the Strang Clinic serving as the clinical division and the institute serving as the research center.

During the past ten years, the focus of the clinic's work has again widened, emphasizing health education and the role of the individual in preventing disease. In this respect, its goal has been to devise lifelong health and safety programs that deter the onset of disease and injury.

Acknowledgments

The staff of the Preventive Medicine Institute/Strang Clinic would like to thank the following consultants for their assistance and valuable suggestions:

Georgia Chavent, M.S., R.D.
Therapeutic Dietitian
Memorial Sloan-Kettering Cancer Center
New York, New York

Ronni Chernoff, Ed.M., R.D.
Clinical Oncology, Research Nutritionist
Department of Surgery
University of Pennsylvania Cancer Center
Philadelphia, Pennsylvania

Isobel Contento, Ph.D.
Associate Professor, Nutrition and Education
Program in Nutrition
Teachers College
Columbia University
New York, New York

Darlene Erlander, M.A., R.D.
Assistant Professor of Nutrition
New York Hospital School of Nursing
New York, New York

Michele Fairchild, M.A., R.D.
Chief Therapeutic Dietitian
Memorial Sloan-Kettering Cancer Center
New York, New York

Judith Wylie, Ed.D., R.D.
Associate in Medicine
Department of Medicine
Albert Einstein College of Medicine
Bronx, New York

We also wish to acknowledge the contributions of Margaret Burbidge, M.S., R.D., Wendy Seda, and Anne Marie Kelly, Preventive Medicine Institute/Strang Clinic.

Introduction

Most of us at one time or another have worried about what and how much we eat, and rightly so. Never before has there been such extensive discussion about nutrition or so many "answers" designed to help us improve our eating habits. Consumers are constantly bombarded with the latest fad diets, nutritional claims, and research findings, which more often confuse than clarify.

Good reasons exist for this state of affairs. In the last few decades rapid and major changes have taken place in our eating habits. Accompanying these changes has been a growing awareness of the impact of nutrition on health. For example, busier life-styles and an increase in the percentage of working women have made the quick meal more popular, even more necessary. Convenience foods, fast-food restaurants, and an abundant food supply have made it all too easy to overeat. We used to worry about getting enough food. Now we worry about eating too much.

In addition to the amount of food within reach, so many of our natural foods have been altered that we are uncertain about the quality and safety of what we eat. Technologies such as refining, freeze-drying, and new methods of preservation have not only made traditional foods more readily available, but have also created "new" foods. Unfortunately, these foods are often highly refined and laden with chemicals that color, flavor, and preserve them. The long-term consequences of a diet high in these foods are as yet unclear, making it difficult to assess the safety of our daily food supply.

As a result of these changes, the American diet, once abundant in fruits, vegetables, and whole grains, is now high in meat, sugar, and refined foods. Our diet has changed from primarily unadulterated foods rich in fiber and nutrients to processed foods high in calories but low in fiber and nutrients. We have lost the variety and balance of whole foods so important for providing the nutrients our bodies require. In other words, we are getting too many calories with too little nutrition.

Along with these changes in dietary habits, there have been gradual shifts in our health problems and disease patterns. The primary focus of medicine is now on chronic diseases such as heart disease, hypertension, diabetes, and cancer. Nutrition is implicated in all of these problems. Although many questions about the role of nutrition in disease remain unanswered, it is already clear that several aspects of our diet are unsound. In general, we consume more calories than we need, too much fat, too much sugar, and too much salt.

Not only are these dietary patterns unhealthy, they are also unnecessary. We have the most abundant and varied food supply in the world; the difficulty is knowing how to eat for good health as well as for pleasure. The Health Action Plan, *Nutrition*, is designed to help you do just that. It will enhance your understanding of your diet as it now exists and will help you to learn how you can improve it. Each topic in this book was specifically chosen because it represents a significant problem area in our current way of eating.

☐ How to use this book

The Health Action Plan, *Nutrition,* is prepared for the average American *adult.* It is not intended for children, pregnant or lactating women, or people requiring therapeutic diets, although many of the principles are generally applicable.

The book is divided into eight parts:

1 **A medical self-assessment**
2 **Calories**
3 **Carbohydrates**
4 **Fats**
5 **Protein**
6 **Sodium**
7 **Vitamins and minerals**
8 **Putting it all together**

Part 1 is a medical self-assessment to help you identify nutritionally related medical problems that may need special attention. Parts 2 through 7 each contain a self-assessment questionnaire to identify areas in your dietary patterns that can be improved. In addition to self-assessment, each section provides important information and guidelines for making changes.

In order to design your personal action plan for improving your diet, record all statements from the self-assessments to which you answer ''no'' in a notebook (see p. 172 for sample). This record outlines the weak areas in your diet. These areas become your goals for change in your personal action plan.

Part 8, ''Putting It All Together,'' serves as a summary. Suggestions in this section will help you select foods for a nutritious diet, devise menus to suit your needs, and prepare foods in an interesting and healthful way.

Before proceeding, we suggest you record your food intake for one week in a small notebook. Be certain to record *everything* you eat or drink, including the amount of each portion of food and the method of preparation. Don't forget snacks. This record will give you a clearer picture of what you actually eat, enabling you to more accurately answer the questions in the self-assessments. Follow the sample on page 171.

As you set out to improve your eating habits, remember that it will take time to make changes. Be persistent, yet patient, and keep in mind that eating is one of the pleasures in life. Enjoy both good health and good eating.

Part 1

Nutrition and your health: a medical self-assessment

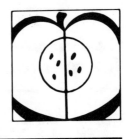

This Health Action Plan, *Nutrition,* is designed for adults considered to be in good health. It is *not* intended for those who have nutritionally related medical problems requiring special attention to diet. Nevertheless, much of the information may be compatible with special diets and may possibly be used in conjunction with recommendations made by your physician and nutritionist. This should be done *only* with their approval, so please check with them before using this plan.

Many of you may be well aware of nutritionally related medical problems you may have, but for some of you, problems may have gone unnoticed or unattended. Consider the following questions to help you identify conditions that may require special attention.

Self-assessment for medical history

I HAVE YOU EVER BEEN TOLD BY A PHYSICIAN THAT YOU HAVE:

	YES	NO
■ Sugar in your urine?	___	___
■ High blood sugar?	___	___
■ An abnormal glucose tolerance?	___	___
■ High blood pressure or hypertension?	___	___
■ Gastric, duodenal, or peptic ulcer?	___	___
■ Elevated cholesterol?	___	___
■ Elevated triglycerides?	___	___
■ A thyroid disorder?	___	___
■ Cancer of the stomach, colon, small intestine, or pancreas?	___	___
■ Anemia?	___	___
■ Decreased kidney function?	___	___
■ Gallbladder disorder?	___	___

The above conditions all have nutritional implications. If you answered "yes" to any of these questions, your nutritional care should be under the guidance of your physician.

II HAVE YOU RECENTLY OR ARE YOU CURRENTLY EXPERIENCING ANY OF THE FOLLOWING:

■ An unexplained weight loss of more than 10 pounds in the last month?	___	___
■ Frequent nausea and/or vomiting?	___	___
■ A change in bowel habits?	___	___

If yes:

		YES	NO
1	Is this change causing frequent constipation?	_____	_____
2	Is this change causing frequent diarrhea?	_____	_____
3	Are you alternating between constipation and diarrhea?	_____	_____

- Tarry black or bloody stools? _____ _____
- Feeling of pins and needles in your hands and/or feet? _____ _____
- Frequent urination (getting up in the middle of the night to urinate)? _____ _____
- Excessive thirst resulting in your drinking more than 8 glasses of fluid a day? _____ _____
- Frequent swelling of your hands and/or ankles? _____ _____
- Frequent pain in ankles or joints? _____ _____

If you answered "yes" to any of these questions, you may have a nutritionally related medical problem that needs special attention. Before continuing with this Health Action Plan, check with your physician about these symptoms.

III HAS ANY BLOOD RELATIVE EVER HAD:

- Diabetes? _____ _____
- Hypertension (high blood pressure)? _____ _____
- Elevated cholesterol and/or triglycerides? _____ _____
- Cancer of the intestine, colon, stomach, or pancreas? _____ _____
- Thyroid disorder? _____ _____

If you answered "yes" to any of these questions, be certain your physician is aware of the family history.

Part 2

Calories: a matter of excess

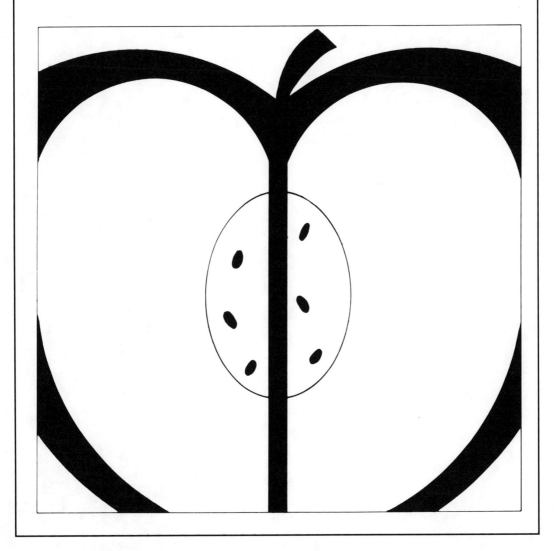

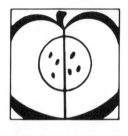

Excessive consumption of calories is one of the most unhealthy and alarming trends in the way Americans eat. In fact, so many unnecessary calories are consumed that an estimated one-third of us are overweight—so overweight that for many life expectancy is shortened.

Most of us know only too well what goes wrong—if more calories are taken into our bodies than are needed, we gain weight. Moreover, excessive intake has been accompanied by a decrease in physical activity. Modern technology, which has given us so many energy-saving devices—automobiles, washing machines, golf carts, electric mixers, power lawn mowers—has also helped remove much of the physical activity that used to be such an integral part of everyday life.

Years of overeating and inactivity inevitably result in steady weight gain—10, 20, 30, or more pounds than we weighed at age twenty is not unusual. While our bodies need fewer calories as we grow older, weight gain does not have to occur. Measures can be taken to assure that added pounds do not accompany added years.

It is only natural to want to shed pounds as quickly and painlessly as possible. Consequently, the market is flooded with all kinds of "quick and easy" diet programs, most of which will indeed result in some temporary weight loss. Our bodies, however, are not designed to function on diets that are all fat, no carbohydrate, all grapefruit, or whatever. In fact, such extreme eating is potentially dangerous because it often results in excesses or deficiencies of important nutrients. Without a *variety* and *balance* of foods we run the risk of poor health.

Moreover, these fad diets are really a way of running away from ourselves—running from eating habits that have been with us for years and will return once the diet is over. Most people manage to follow such diets for only a few weeks anyway and then experience a discouraging, rapid weight gain, because they return to their former eating patterns.

It is possible to lose weight and keep it off only by making *permanent* changes in eating habits. Such changes require an understanding of why and how we overeat and what we can do to make lasting changes.

Many people are not aware of the habits that put on those extra pounds. If you find yourself heavier than you would like to be, you probably need to make changes in the intake of sugar and fats in your diet. (See Part 3, "Carbohydrates: Heroes or Villains," and Part 4, "Fat: The Controversial Nutrient.") Excess empty calories from fats, sugar, and alcohol are leading offenders. Put them in balance and you may discover that you have conquered your weight problem.

In addition to specific food choices, eating behavior greatly influences total calories consumed each day. Many people take in extra calories by using food to deal with anxiety, stress, boredom, anger, or fatigue. Eating compulsively or rapidly while watching TV or reading is another habit that can lead to overeating.

Weight control is very individual. For some it comes naturally; for others it is a matter of being more aware of those extra calories or of modifying behavior that often results in overeating.

Facts to consider

- Obesity is one of the most serious nutritional problems in America today.

- An estimated 15,000,000 Americans are obese to the extent that their health is in jeopardy.

- Obesity is associated with the onset and progression of hypertension, diabetes, heart disease, and gallbladder disease.

- Our sedentary life-style is considered a contributing factor in the incidence of overweight in this country. Physical exercise is important for maintaining an ideal body weight and good muscle tone.

- As we grow older, we require fewer calories to maintain an ideal body weight.

- Identifying and changing eating behavior are often the keys to permanent weight control.

- Many people overeat by eating too fast.

- Skipping meals during the day often results in evening binges.

- Many people overeat by using food to deal with anxieties, frustrations, and boredom.

- Regular exercise not only uses up excess calories but also can help relieve tensions that often lead to overeating.

Weight chart of persons twenty years and older

MEN

HEIGHT (without shoes)	WEIGHT (without clothing)	
	Normal range	Obesity level*
5'3"	118–141	169
5'4"	122–145	174
5'5"	126–149	179
5'6"	130–155	186
5'7"	134–161	193
5'8"	139–166	199
5'9"	143–170	204
5'10"	147–174	209
5'11"	150–178	214
6'0"	154–183	220
6'1"	158–188	226
6'2"	162–192	230
6'3"	165–195	234

WOMEN

5'0"	100–118	142
5'1"	104–121	145
5'2"	107–125	150
5'3"	110–128	154
5'4"	113–132	158
5'5"	116–135	162
5'6"	120–139	167
5'7"	123–142	170
5'8"	126–146	175
5'9"	130–151	181
5'10"	133–156	187
5'11"	137–161	193
6'0"	141–166	199

*A weight above 20% of upper normal is generally considered the obesity level.
Adapted from: U.S. Department of Agriculture, Home and Garden Bulletin No. 74.

Self-assessment
for calories

To help you assess your calorie intake, answer the following questions about body weight, food choices, and eating behavior. Record all statements to which you answer "no" in your notebook, following the sample on page 172. When the action plan is completed, you will have a personal outline for eating patterns that need changing.

☐ Body weight

DO YOU:

	YES	NO
■ Maintain your weight within a normal range for your height? (See chart, page 11.)	_____	_____
■ Watch that your weight does not increase as you grow older?	_____	_____
■ Avoid large swings in weight gain or weight loss (more than 15 pounds at a time)?	_____	_____

☐ Food choices

DO YOU USUALLY:

	YES	NO
■ Limit the amount of sugar you eat? (See Part 3, "Carbohydrates.")	_____	_____
■ Limit the amount of fat in your diet? (See Part 4, "Fats.")	_____	_____
■ Know the calorie content of foods you eat regularly?	_____	_____
■ Limit the size of your food portions?	_____	_____
■ Limit alcohol consumption to an average of not more than one drink per day? (One drink equals 1 jigger—1$^1/_2$ ounces—of hard liquor, a 4-ounce glass of wine, or a 12-ounce can of beer.)	_____	_____
■ Limit or avoid high-calorie snacks such as cookies, sodas, nuts, chips, or candy?	_____	_____
■ Avoid diet crazes such as the liquid protein diet, the no-carbohydrate diet, or the grapefruit diet?	_____	_____

☐ Eating behavior

DO YOU USUALLY:

	YES	NO
■ Eat slowly (take at least twenty minutes to eat a meal)?	_____	_____
■ Take only one portion of food at a meal?	_____	_____
■ Avoid going for long periods without eating?	_____	_____
■ When bored, find activities other than eating to break the boredom?	_____	_____
■ Deal with anger in ways that do not involve eating?	_____	_____
■ Find ways of dealing with fatigue other than eating?	_____	_____
■ Have ways for dealing with anxiety that do not involve eating?	_____	_____
■ Avoid other activities while eating, such as reading, watching television, working in the kitchen?	_____	_____
■ Know your "danger" periods during the day when you are likely to overeat?	_____	_____
■ Know which foods you have a tendency to overeat?	_____	_____
■ Avoid stocking up on "problem foods" for "unexpected guests"?	_____	_____
■ Confine your eating, including snacks, to one location in the house?	_____	_____
■ Avoid eating food off the plates of others, such as when feeding children or when cleaning up?	_____	_____
■ Buy and prepare only the amount of food you need?	_____	_____
■ Avoid eating after dinner?	_____	_____

☐ Making changes

Now that you have learned something about your eating patterns, you are in a position to make some changes. Let the following guide help you to reduce and control body weight.

CONTROL WEIGHT BY INCREASING ACTIVITY

It is as simple as that: you can help control weight by increasing physical activity. Generally you can do this in two ways.

First, and most important, increase physical activity in your everyday routine. For example, try walking instead of driving or riding. Walk at least part of the way to work, to run errands, or to shop. Get into the habit of using stairs instead of elevators. Participate in sports instead of always being the spectator. Think about your daily routine and devise as many ways as you can to increase physical activity.

Next, devise an exercise program and work at it regularly (see the Health Action Plan, *Physical Fitness*). You might join a gym or exercise club, run, jog, dance, or play tennis. No matter what activities you enjoy, the important thing is to exercise regularly.

TUNE IN TO CALORIES

Extra weight may have sneaked up on you simply because you have not paid attention to extra calories in your diet. Don't despair. You probably will not find it difficult to shed those pounds once you are "tuned into" your calorie consumption.

No matter how you look at it, calories do count. That doesn't mean that you must spend tedious hours calculating your diet down to the last morsel. But you do need to know where the calories come from and how to control your intake of them.

It's all a matter of supply and demand. Consider the following facts:

- You will *lose* weight if you take in fewer food calories than your body's energy demand. Your body will use its own stored fat to make up the deficit.

- You will *maintain* your weight if you supply your body with just enough food calories to meet its energy demand.

- You will *gain* weight if you take in more food calories than your body's energy demand. Your body will store the excess energy as fat.

Now, think about the following statements. Begin to consider some of the eating habits that might be putting on extra pounds. For example, did you know that:

- If you drink a lot of tea and coffee with sugar, you may be adding several hundred calories to your diet each day?

- By eating lean meats instead of fatty meats, you can cut hundreds of calories from your diet each day?

- A mixed drink such as gin and tonic may have as many as 200 calories while a glass of dry wine may have as little as 85?

As you can see, calories can sneak up on you in many different ways. Start paying attention to the calorie contents of the foods you eat. With a bit of "tuning in," you'll soon be cutting down naturally.

**BROWSE THROUGH A
CALORIE CHART**
One way to "tune into" calories is to study a calorie chart. Look through the calorie chart beginning on page 29. You may be amazed to discover that foods you thought were low in calories are in fact high, while other foods you always thought were high in calories are really relatively low.

For example, did you know that:

- An avocado has nearly 400 calories, or that an apple has nearly as many calories as a banana?

- One-half cup of raisins has as many as 240 calories, while 1 cup of popcorn without butter or oil has as few as 40?

- Bread and potatoes aren't really so bad: only 90 calories in an average boiled potato and 65 in a slice of bread?

Obviously, some foods we consider to be healthful—avocados and raisins—are higher in calories than expected, while foods we consider fattening—bread and popcorn—are lower. Often it is how we prepare certain foods that makes them high in calories. Putting mayonnaise on a slice of bread, sour cream on a potato, or butter on popcorn can make their calorie contents soar! Also, watch out for those extra calories that salad dressings and oils contribute. Take a look at the calories in the foods you eat regularly and also consider what you add to them when you eat them. You might find it rewarding to think of ways to eat foods you love and still cut down on extra calories.

**WATCH OUT FOR THE FATS
IN YOUR DIET**
Fats are discussed in detail in Part 4, but for now it is important to emphasize that fats have more than twice the calories of proteins or carbohydrates. Moreover, fats have a way of creeping into your diet without your realizing it. Be aware that you can save many calories in the following ways:

- Eat lean meats instead of fatty meats.

- Cook meats on a rack so that the fat can drip off the meat and into a pan.

- Trim all fat off meats. Hundreds of calories can be saved by eating fat-trimmed or lean meats.

- Avoid or cut down on fried foods. For example, you can save 135 calories by having a baked potato instead of hash browns.

- Buy water-packed instead of oil-packed tuna, or drain and rinse oil from canned fish.

- Avoid cream or creamers in coffee and tea. Use milk, preferably skimmed. You can save 14 calories per tablespoon.

- Drink skim or low-fat milk instead of whole milk. By using skim milk, you will cut calories in half.

- Avoid gravies. Most gravy is made with meat fat. Instead, season food with herbs and spices.

- Eat broth soups instead of cream soups. This would mean a saving of approximately 80 calories per cup.

- Use low-fat—or just less—salad dressing. There are many low-calorie salad dressings available; even better, try seasoning salads with lemon juice.

- Cut down or eliminate high-fat spreads on breads and rolls. Watch out for butter, margarine, or mayonnaise, all of which are high in fat. Be aware that diet margarines and imitation mayonnaises have half the calories of the regular products.

- Avoid or limit high-fat desserts. High-fat desserts include pies, ice cream, custards, and most cakes.

- Avoid high-fat snacks such as potato chips and nuts.

LIMIT THE AMOUNT OF SUGAR IN YOUR DIET

Sugar is discussed in detail in Part 3, but for the moment remember that sugar and high-sugar products are high in calories. Review the points made in Part 3 and keep in mind the following suggestions.

- Learn to drink unsweetened or less-sweetened coffee or tea. For each teaspoon eliminated you can save 20 to 40 calories, depending on how high you heap sugar on the spoon.

- Avoid sweet drinks such as soft drinks and fruit drinks. One can of soda adds 145 calories to your diet.

- Eat fresh or water-packed fruit. Fruit packed in syrup is high in calories. If you do buy such fruit, drain or rinse it before serving.

- Be aware that dried fruits are high in sugar calories.

- Choose cereals that are low in sugar. Read labels before selecting cereal products (see page 61).

- Avoid or limit your intake of candies and sweet desserts.

- Be aware that many processed foods have added sugar. Processed foods such as ketchup, peanut butter, cold cuts, vegetables, and cereals often have added sugar. Read labels and whenever possible select foods without added sugar.

LEARN TO CALORIE-SUBSTITUTE

Become aware of how easy it is to pick up extra calories without thinking. Eliminate these excess calories from your diet by substituting low-calorie foods for high-calorie foods. Reducing excess calories is really quite easy. It is only a matter of learning where you can cut down on unwanted calories and where you will miss them least.

The daily menu on the next page shows how a typical "uncontrolled" diet can be trimmed by almost 3,000 "hidden" calories.

Daily menu substitution

BREAKFAST

FROM	Calories	TO	Calories	Calories saved
½ glass (4 oz) orange juice	56	½ glass (4 oz) orange juice	56	0
¾ cup granola-type cereal	375	¾ cup Bran Flakes	80	295
½ cup whole milk	80	½ cup skim milk	44	36
1 cup coffee with:	0	1 cup coffee with:	0	0
2 tsp sugar	30	no sugar	0	30
2 tbsp cream	64	2 tbsp skim milk	11	53
Total	**605**	**Total**	**191**	**414**

MID-MORNING SNACK

FROM	Calories	TO	Calories	Calories saved
1 Danish pastry	275	2 graham crackers	55	220
1 cup coffee with:	0	1 cup coffee with:	0	0
2 tsp sugar	30	no sugar	0	30
2 tbsp cream	64	2 tbsp skim milk	11	53
Total	**369**	**Total**	**66**	**303**

LUNCH

FROM	Calories	TO	Calories	Calories saved
2 oz bologna	172	2 oz chicken (white)	94	78
2 slices white bread	150	2 slices whole-wheat melba thin bread	75	75
1 tbsp mayonnaise	101	1 tbsp low-calorie mayonnaise	50	51
1 glass (8 oz) whole milk	160	1 glass (8 oz) skim milk	88	72
1 slice chocolate cake with icing	235	1 small banana	85	150
Total	**818**	**Total**	**392**	**426**

MID-AFTERNOON SNACK

FROM	Calories	TO	Calories	Calories saved
1 can (12 oz) cola	150	12 oz club soda	0	150
3 chocolate chip cookies	155	3 vanilla wafers	42	113
Total	**305**	**Total**	**42**	**263**

DINNER

FROM	Calories	TO	Calories	Calories saved
1 cup cream of mushroom soup	216	1 cup chicken rice soup	48	168
6 oz meat loaf	680	4 oz broiled flank steak	220	460
with 4 tbsp gravy	164	no gravy	0	164
½ cup scalloped potatoes (with cheese)	178	½ cup mashed potatoes	99	79
12 asparagus spears	40	12 asparagus spears	40	0
2 dinner rolls with:	170	2 small slices whole-wheat Italian bread with:	88	82
2 tsp butter	70	2 tsp diet margarine	34	36
Hearts of lettuce with:	20	Hearts of lettuce with:	20	0
½ tbsp dressing	115	1½ tbsp low-calorie dressing	18	97
Apple pie	300	Baked apple	120	180
1 cup coffee with:	0	1 cup coffee with:	0	0
2 tsp sugar	30	no sugar	0	30
2 tbsp cream	64	2 tbsp skim milk	11	53
Total	**2047**	**Total**	**698**	**1349**
Total for day	**4144**	**Total for day**	**1389**	**2755**

Calorie substitutions

Review the following suggestions for calorie substitutions. Note any food that you eat at least once a month. In the future, plan to substitute the lower-calorie food suggested in the column on the right, or select another low-calorie substitution from the calorie chart that begins on page 29.

BEVERAGES

INSTEAD OF THIS	Calories	HAVE THIS	Calories	Calories saved
Whole milk—8 oz	160	Skim milk—8 oz	90	70
Prune juice—4 oz	100	Tomato juice—4 oz	25	75
Soft drink—12 oz	144	Iced tea—12 oz, unsweetened	0	144
Coffee—1 cup with:	0	Coffee—1 cup with:	0	0
Sugar—2 tsp	30	No sugar	0	30
Cream—2 tbsp	64	Skim milk—1 tbsp	11	53
Chocolate malted milk—8 oz	500	Low-fat chocolate milk drink—8 oz	77	423
Grape juice—8 oz	170	Grapefruit juice—8 oz	100	70
Tom Collins—6 oz Collins and 1½ oz gin	195	Dry white wine—4 oz	88	107

MEATS (COOKED)

Porterhouse steak—4 oz	527	Flank steak—4 oz	222	305
Hamburger, regular—4 oz	327	Hamburger, lean ground round—4 oz	247	80
Ribs of beef—4 oz	499	Round roast—4 oz	220	279
Loin lamb chops—4 oz	407	Leg of lamb roast, trimmed—4 oz	211	196
Spareribs—4 oz	499	Pork center loin chop, trimmed—4 oz	288	211
Bacon—2 strips	85	Canadian bacon—1 slice	60	25
Shoulder lamb chop—4 oz	380	Loin lamb chop, trimmed—4 oz	206	174

FISH AND POULTRY

INSTEAD OF THIS	Calories	HAVE THIS	Calories	Calories saved
Roasted duck—4 oz	**413**	Roasted chicken—4 oz	**213**	**200**
Tuna, oil-packed, drained—4 oz	**224**	Tuna, water-packed—4 oz	**144**	**80**
Pickled marinated herring—4 oz	**252**	Canned herring in tomato sauce—4 oz	**200**	**52**
Lobster meat—4 oz with 2 tbsp butter	**300**	Lobster meat—4 oz with lemon	**95**	**205**

SANDWICHES

	Calories		Calories	Calories saved
2 oz bologna with 1 tbsp mayo	**423**	2 oz white meat chicken or turkey with 1 tbsp low-cal mayo	**294**	**129**
Cheeseburger—3 oz with bun	**411**	Hamburger—3 oz open-face	**246**	**165**
2 oz liverwurst	**330**	Lean roast beef—2 oz	**267**	**63**
Club (3 slices bread, turkey—2 oz, bacon— 2 slices, mayo—2 tbsp)	**612**	Turkey—2 oz with tomato, low-cal mayo—1 tbsp, 1 slice bread	**250**	**362**
Egg salad on roll, 2 tbsp mayo	**440**	Egg salad open-face, low-cal mayo—2 tbsp	**258**	**182**
Grilled cheese—2 oz	**430**	Cottage cheese—¼ cup, tomato	**210**	**220**

SALADS

	Calories		Calories	Calories saved
½ avocado with 1 tbsp mayo	**305**	Marinated asparagus— 6 stalks	**40**	**265**
Marinated 3-bean salad— ½ cup	**337**	Pickled beet salad—½ cup	**43**	**294**
Tossed salad with 2 tbsp Roquefort or blue cheese	**192**	Tossed salad with 1 tbsp low-cal dressing	**52**	**140**
Spinach salad with 3 strips bacon and 2 tbsp creamy dressing	**308**	Spinach salad—no bacon, 2 tbsp low-cal French dressing	**60**	**248**

Calorie substitutions
(continued)

SOUPS

INSTEAD OF THIS	Calories	HAVE THIS	Calories	Calories saved
Cream of chicken with milk—1 cup	180	Cream of chicken with water—1 cup	95	85
New England clam chowder—1 cup	203	Manhattan clam chowder—1 cup	80	123
French onion soup—1 cup with cheese (2 oz) and bread	340	Plain onion soup—1 cup	65	275

VEGETABLES

Hashed brown potatoes—1 cup	350	Baked potato—1 medium	145	205
French fries—10 strips	215	Boiled potato—½ cup, 1 tsp low-cal margarine	71	144
Baked·beans—½ cup	153	Green beans—½ cup	15	138
Peas—½ cup	65	Asparagus—4 stalks	14	51
Winter squash—½ cup	45	Summer squash—½ cup	15	30
Beets—½ cup	30	Cauliflower—½ cup	15	15

CHEESES, SPREADS, DRESSINGS

Butter or margarine—1 tsp or 1 pat	35	Diet margarine—1 tsp	17	18
Mayo—1 tbsp	100	Imitation mayo—1 tbsp	55	45
Creamy salad dressing—1 tbsp	76	Low-cal salad dressing—1 tbsp	15	61
Oil and vinegar—1 tbsp	80	Lemon juice—1 tbsp	3	77

SNACKS

INSTEAD OF THIS	Calories	HAVE THIS	Calories	Calories saved
Chocolate chip cookies—3 (1¾" diam)	103	Whole-wheat crackers—3	66	37
Dry roasted peanuts—½ cup	425	Dry roasted soynuts—½ cup	195	230
Roasted cashews—½ cup	393	Apple—1 med	96	297
Potato chips—10 med	114	Pretzel sticks—10 sticks (3½" x ⅛")	23	91

DESSERTS

Ice cream—½ cup	129	Yogurt (plain)—½ cup	75	54
Cheesecake—2" piece	200	Sponge cake—2" piece	120	80
Chocolate cake with icing—1 slice	425	Banana bread—1 slice	119	306
Apple pie—⅛ pie	300	Baked apple	120	180
Pecan pie—⅛ pie	431	Fresh strawberries—1 cup	55	376

CONSIDER PORTION SIZES

Learn to be aware of the size of your portions. Measure and weigh foods until you are sure you can accurately judge portions. Eating smaller amounts of the same foods can make a big difference.

FROM	TO	CALORIES SAVED
3 tbsp peanut butter	1$\frac{1}{2}$ tbsp	**150**
$\frac{1}{2}$ lb hamburger	$\frac{1}{4}$ lb hamburger*	**240**
8 oz steak	4 oz steak*	**250**
2 eggs	1 egg	**90**
1 cup rice	$\frac{1}{2}$ cup rice	**110**
1 cup spaghetti	$\frac{1}{2}$ cup spaghetti	**75**
2 slices bread	1 slice bread	**65**

*See pages 99–103 for guidelines to meat portions.

TIPS FOR CONTROLLING APPETITE

In addition to becoming aware of the number of calories you regularly eat, it helps to learn a few ways to control your appetite so that cutting down portions will be easier. If you find that in taking steps to control calories you feel hungry, try the following methods.

- Start each meal with a filling, but low-calorie, appetizer. For example, have clear soup or broth, a few celery sticks or other raw vegetable, or a small green salad with low-fat dressing.

- Drink a glass of cold water or cold, low-salt club soda with lemon. A cold drink helps to curb hunger pangs.

- Eat a small portion of a carbohydrate food about a half hour before your meal. If you find that you are too hungry at mealtime, try having one or two soda crackers, a small glass of vegetable juice, or half a grapefruit before the main meal. This may help curb your appetite and allow you to eat less. Eating solid food results in a much greater sense of fullness than drinking liquids. Solid foods stay in the stomach longer and cause a stretching of the stomach wall, thus contributing to a sense of satiety.

- Use vegetables to provide low-calorie bulk to a meal.

CONTROLLING CALORIES WHEN EATING OUT

As difficult as it is to control calories when you eat out, there are a few tricks for reducing calories. Keep the following guidelines in mind.

BREAD

Ask to have the bread, rolls, and butter removed from the table. If you avoid a pre-meal plunge into the bread, many calories will be saved. If you are with guests who want to have the bread, try keeping it on the opposite side of the table or cover it so that it is out of sight.

APPETIZERS AND SOUP
Choose fresh fruits, fruit juices, broth-based soups, and seafood (except those fried or in cream sauces).

ENTREES
Choose meats that are broiled, roasted, or baked.

Select low-fat meat such as seafood, chicken or turkey (without skin), veal, and beef such as London broil or tenderloin. Ask to have fish and meats cooked without butter, or at least leave most of the butter or sauce on your plate. Always ask about ingredients when uncertain from the description on the menu. If portions are large, save calories by eating half of what is served.

VEGETABLES
Choose vegetables that are plain (without sauce). Save calories by limiting or avoiding sour cream and butter. Limit higher-calorie vegetables such as potatoes, corn, and peas.

SALADS
Ask that dressings be served on the side so that you control the amount used (or even better, use lemon juice or vinegar). Avoid high-calorie ingredients such as croutons, bacon, cheese, avocado.

SANDWICHES
Ask that spreads such as mayonnaise, butter, margarine, and other dressings be served on the side so that you control the amounts used. Mustard, lettuce, tomatoes, and toasted bread improve sandwiches without adding the calories of spreads.

Choose lower-calorie fillings such as lean beef, chicken, turkey, tuna, sliced egg.

Having an open-face sandwich eliminates the calories of an extra slice of bread.

BEVERAGES
Try having ice water or club soda with meals—it is refreshing and filling with no calories.

Cultivate a taste for tea and coffee without sugar or cream.

If having an alcoholic beverage, limit yourself to one cocktail on the rocks or mixed with water or club soda, or one glass of *dry* wine.

DESSERTS
Choose fresh fruits.

Be aware of the high-calorie cost of pies, cakes, ice cream, and so on. If you are going to have these items occasionally, plan to limit the calories elsewhere. Avoiding a la modes, whipped cream, and frosting helps reduce calories.

LIMIT CALORIES BY CHANGING EATING BEHAVIOR

In addition to specific food choices, many other aspects of eating behavior influence how much we eat. Changing these habits isn't always easy, but it can be done. Become aware of your habits and let the following techniques help you to make changes.

ALLOW AT LEAST TWENTY MINUTES TO EAT A MEAL

It takes approximately twenty minutes after food has reached your stomach for the brain to get the message that enough food has been eaten. Eating too fast is likely to result in overeating. To slow down:

- Take a three- to five-minute rest period midway in the meal.
- Pay more attention to the taste, smell, and texture of the food.
- Try to be the last person to finish each course of a meal.
- Cut food into small pieces.
- Put down your fork between bites, or between every second or third bite.

DO NOT SKIP MEALS OR GO LONG PERIODS WITHOUT EATING

Regular meals and small snacks allow you to control extreme hunger that so often results in binge eating. For example, skipping breakfast and lunch is likely to result in an evening of constant eating. Plan to eat every three to five hours.

INSTEAD OF EATING WHEN YOU ARE BORED:

- Engage in other pleasurable activities.
- Call or visit a supportive friend.
- Take up a hobby or special project.
- Get out of the house.
- Consider possibilities such as community activities and courses at a local school.

**INSTEAD OF EATING
WHEN YOU ARE ANGRY, TRY:**

- Putting your feelings down on paper while you are still angry; analyze the situation to see what made you angry.

- Expressing your feelings directly to the person involved.

- Talking about it with a supportive friend.

- Diverting your attention to a pleasurable activity or thought.

- Chewing gum.

**INSTEAD OF EATING WHEN
YOU ARE FEELING FATIGUED:**

When people are very tired they often eat in order to "get more energy." Don't let fatigue be a problem for you. Plan how you will handle this situation.

- Be certain to get enough sleep. Sleep regular hours and get enough to keep you going comfortably.

- Take a relaxing shower or bath.

- Take a few moments to relax. Drink a cool, low-calorie beverage such as club soda with lemon or iced tea.

- Perk up by getting some fresh air, taking a brisk walk, or doing some exercise.

**INSTEAD OF EATING WHEN
YOU ARE ANXIOUS, TRY:**

- Dealing with the problem causing the anxiety.

- Engaging in physical activity or other enjoyable pastimes.

- Diverting your attention from the problem by thinking about something that pleases you.

**AVOID EATING FOOD OFF
THE PLATES OF OTHER PEOPLE**

Be aware when you do this, especially when clearing the table or cleaning up after a meal. *Stop it!* Scrape the food directly into the garbage. You are not going to save the starving people of the world by eating the scraps. Try buying less food, preparing less, and serving smaller portions.

**AVOID EATING SNACKS
WITH THE CHILDREN**

This is often a problem, especially with foods like cookies, cakes, and other sweets. Neither you nor the children need these foods. Try serving fruit, graham crackers, or soynuts. If you enjoy eating with them, plan your snack to coincide with theirs. Consider ways to avoid snacks, control snacks, or control what you have as a snack. For example, prepare snacks ahead of time, then bring them out only when the children are ready to eat.

GET "PROBLEM FOODS" UNDER CONTROL

Many of us have special "problem foods" that are hard to resist, such as peanuts, chocolate, cookies, and potato chips. To keep calories down, learn what your problem foods are so that they can be controlled. List those foods that give you trouble and record how you are going to control them. Are you going to:

- Avoid them?

- Restrict how often you eat them?

- Control the portion size?

DON'T KEEP "PROBLEM FOODS" JUST IN CASE THERE ARE GUESTS

Stop fooling yourself! This excuse often results in a constant temptation that can't be resisted. If you feel that you must maintain a supply, buy food that you don't particularly like to eat. Store these foods out of sight and out of easy reach.

AVOID ENGAGING IN OTHER ACTIVITIES WHILE EATING

You may have learned to be hungry while doing other things. For example, you may have conditioned yourself to feel hungry while watching TV or when reading a book or newspaper. For some people this is a dangerous habit, since it is easy to be unaware of what and how much you are eating. Recondition this response by eating without distraction. For example:

- Don't have food near while watching TV.

- Engage in some activity during commercials such as exercising, sewing or knitting, talking with someone, or skimming the newspaper.

- Avoid reading while eating.

The suggestions given to help you to reduce your calories and control your weight are designed to help you change your eating patterns and behavior. Only by understanding these patterns, planning to change them, and making the changes can you begin to gain control. Control over your eating behavior will result in permanent weight control.

Calorie chart

BEVERAGES (not including milk beverages and fruit juices)

		Number of calories			Number of calories
CARBONATED BEVERAGES			**Wines:**		
Ginger ale	8 oz glass	75	Table wines (such as Chablis, claret, Rhine wine, and sauterne)	1 small wine glass (about 3½ oz)	85
	12 oz can or bottle	115			
Cola-type	8 oz glass	95	Dessert wines (such as muscatel, port, sherry, and Tokay)	1 small wine glass (about 3½ oz)	140
	12 oz can or bottle	145			
Fruit flavored soda	8 oz glass	115			
	12 oz can or bottle	170	**FRUIT DRINKS, CANNED**		
Root beer	8 oz glass	100	Apricot nectar	½ cup	70
	12 oz can or bottle	150	Cranberry juice cocktail, canned	½ cup	80
ALCOHOLIC BEVERAGES			Grape drink	½ cup	70
Beer, 3.6 percent alcohol by weight	12 oz can	150	Lemonade, frozen concentrate, sweetened, diluted, ready-to-serve	½ cup	55
Whisky, gin, rum, vodka:			Orange juice–apricot juice drink	½ cup	60
100 proof	1 jigger (1½ oz)	125	Peach nectar	½ cup	60
90 proof	1 jigger (1½ oz)	110	Pear nectar	½ cup	65
86 proof	1 jigger (1½ oz)	105	Pineapple juice–grapefruit juice drink	½ cup	70
80 proof	1 jigger (1½ oz)	95	Pineapple juice–orange juice drink	½ cup	70

BREAD AND CEREALS

		Number of calories			Number of calories
BREAD			White:		
			Soft crumb:		
Cracked wheat	1 slice, 9/16″ thick	65	Regular slice	1 slice, 9/16″ thick	70
Raisin	1 slice, ½″ thick	65	Thin slice	1 slice, 7/16″ thick	55
Rye	1 slice, 7/16″ thick	60	Firm crumb	1 slice 7/16″ thick	65

Calorie chart (continued)

		Number of calories
Whole wheat:		
Soft crumb	1 slice, $^9/_{16}$″ thick	65
Firm crumb	1 slice, $^9/_{16}$″ thick	60

CEREALS AND PASTAS

		Number of calories
Bran flakes (40 percent bran)	1 oz (about $^4/_5$ cup)	85
Bran flakes with raisins	1 oz (about $^3/_5$ cup)	80
Corn, puffed, presweetened	1 oz (about 1 cup)	115
Corn, shredded	1 oz (about 1$^1/_6$ cups)	110
Corn flakes	1 oz (about 1$^1/_6$ cups)	110
Corn flakes, sugar coated	1 oz (about $^2/_3$ cup)	110
Corn grits, degermed, cooked	$^3/_4$ cup	95
Farina, cooked, quick-cooking	$^3/_4$ cup	80
Macaroni, cooked	$^3/_4$ cup	115
Macaroni and cheese:		
Home recipe	$^1/_2$ cup	215
Canned	$^1/_2$ cup	115
Noodles, cooked	$^3/_4$ cup	150
Oats, puffed	1 oz (about 1$^1/_6$ cups)	115
Oats, puffed, sugar coated	1 oz (about $^4/_5$ cup)	115
Oatmeal or rolled oats, cooked	$^3/_4$ cup	100
Rice, puffed	1 oz (about 2 cups)	115
Rice, puffed, presweetened	1 oz (about $^2/_3$ cup)	110
Rice, shredded	1 oz (about 1$^1/_8$ cups)	115

		Number of calories
Rice flakes	1 oz (about 1 cup)	110
Spaghetti, cooked	$^3/_4$ cup	115
Spaghetti with meat balls:		
Home recipe	$^3/_4$ cup	250
Canned	$^3/_4$ cup	195
Spaghetti in tomato sauce with cheese:		
Home recipe	$^3/_4$ cup	195
Canned	$^3/_4$ cup	140
Wheat, puffed	1 oz (about 1$^7/_8$ cups)	105
Wheat, puffed, presweetened	1 oz (about $^4/_5$ cup)	105
Wheat, rolled, cooked	$^3/_4$ cup	135
Wheat, shredded, plain (long, round, or bite-size)	1 oz (1 large biscuit or $^1/_2$ cup bite-size)	100
Wheat flakes	1 oz (about 1 cup)	100

DOUGHNUTS

		Number of calories
Cake-type, plain	1 doughnut, 3$^1/_4$″ diam	165
Yeast-leavened, raised	1 doughnut, 3$^3/_4$″ diam	175

MUFFINS

		Number of calories
Plain	1 muffin, 3″ diam	120
Blueberry	1 muffin, 2$^3/_8$″ diam	110
Bran	1 muffin, 2$^5/_8$″ diam	105
Corn	1 muffin, 2$^3/_8$″ diam	125

PANCAKES (GRIDDLE CAKES)

		Number of calories
Wheat (home recipe or mix)	1 cake, 4″ diam	60

		Number of calories				Number of calories
Buckwheat	1 cake, 4″ diam	**55**		Vanilla wafer	1 cookie, 1¾″ diam	**20**
Waffles	1 waffle, 7″ diam	**210**		Custard, baked	½ cup	**150**
				Gelatin desserts, ready-to-serve:		
DESSERTS				Plain	½ cup	**70**
				Fruit added	½ cup	**80**
Apple betty	½ cup	**160**		Ice, fruit	½ cup	**125**
Brownie, with nuts	1 piece, 1¾″ square, ⅞″ thick	**90**		Ice cream, plain:		
				Regular	½ cup	**130**
				Rich	½ cup	**165**
Cakes:				Ice milk:		
Angel food cake	2½″ sector (1/12 of a 9¾″ round cake)	**135**		Hardened	½ cup	**100**
				Soft serve	½ cup	**135**
Butter cake:				Pies:		
Plain, without icing	1 piece, 3″ x 3″ x 2″	**315**		Apple	3½″ sector (⅛ of 9″ pie)	**300**
	1 cupcake, 2¾″ diam	**115**		Blueberry	3½″ sector (⅛ of 9″ pie)	**285**
Plain, with chocolate icing	1¾″ sector (1/16 of 9″ round layer cake)	**240**		Cherry	3½″ sector (⅛ of 9″ pie)	**310**
	1 cupcake, 2¾″ diam	**170**		Chocolate meringue	3½″ sector (⅛ of 9″ pie)	**285**
Chocolate, with chocolate icing	1¾″ sector (1/16 of 9″ round layer cake)	**235**		Coconut custard	3½″ sector (⅛ of 9″ pie)	**270**
Fruitcake, dark	1 piece, 2″ x 1½″ x ¼″	**55**		Custard	3½″ sector (⅛ of 9″ pie)	**250**
Gingerbread	1 piece, 2¾″ x 2¾″ x 1⅜″	**175**		Lemon meringue	3½″ sector (⅛ of 9″ pie)	**270**
Pound cake, old-fashioned	1 slice, 3½″ x 3″ x ½″	**140**		Mince	3½″ sector (⅛ of 9″ pie)	**320**
Sponge cake	1⅞″ sector (1/16 of 9¾″ round cake)	**145**		Peach	3½″ sector (⅛ of 9″ pie)	**300**
Cookies:				Pecan	3½″ sector (⅛ of 9″ pie)	**430**
Chocolate chip	1 cookie, 2⅓″ diam, ½″ thick	**50**		Pumpkin	3½″ sector (⅛ of 9″ pie)	**240**
Fig bars, small	1 fig bar	**50**		Raisin	3½″ sector (⅛ of 9″ pie)	**320**
Sandwich, chocolate or vanilla	1 cookie, 1¾″ diam, ⅜″ thick	**50**				
Sugar	1 cookie, 2¼″ diam	**35**				

Calorie chart (continued)

		Number of calories			Number of calories
Rhubarb	3½" sector (⅛ of 9" pie)	300	Cheese	1 cracker, 2" diam	15
Strawberry	3½" sector (⅛ of 9" pie)	185	Graham	1 med	28
Prune whip	½ cup	70	Saltines	1 cracker, 1⅞" square	13
Puddings:			Oyster	10 crackers	35
Cornstarch	½ cup	140	Rye	1 wafer, 1⅞" x 3½"	23
Chocolate, from a mix	½ cup	160	Pizza (cheese)	5⅓" sector, ⅛ of a 13¾" pie	155
Rennet desserts, ready-to-serve	½ cup	115	Pretzels:		
Tapioca cream	½ cup	110	Dutch, twisted	1 pretzel	60
Sherbet	½ cup	130	Stick	5 regular (3⅛" long) or 10 small (2¼" long)	10
OTHER BAKED GOODS			Rolls:		
Baking powder biscuit:			Danish pastry, plain	1 pastry, 4½" diam	275
Home recipe	1 biscuit, 2" diam	105	Hamburger or frankfurter	1 roll (16 per pound)	120
Mix	1 biscuit, 2" diam	90	Hard, round or rectangular	1 roll (9 per pound)	155
Crackers:			Plain, pan	1 roll (16 per pound)	85
Butter	1 cracker, 2" diam	15			

FATS, OILS, AND RELATED PRODUCTS

Butter or margarine	1 tbsp	100	**SALAD DRESSINGS**		
	1 pat (1 tsp), 1" square, ⅓" thick	35	Regular:		
			French	1 tbsp	65
			Blue cheese	1 tbsp	75
			Home-cooked, boiled	1 tbsp	25
Margarine, whipped	1 tbsp	70	Italian	1 tbsp	85
	1 pat (1 tsp), 1¼" square, ⅓" thick	25	Mayonnaise	1 tbsp	100
			Salad dressing, commercial, plain (mayonnaise-type)	1 tbsp	65
Cooking fats:			Russian	1 tbsp	75
Vegetable	1 tbsp	110	Thousand Island	1 tbsp	80
Lard	1 tbsp	115	Low calorie:		
Salad or cooking oils	1 tbsp	120	French	1 tbsp	15
			Italian	1 tbsp	10
			Thousand Island	1 tbsp	25

GRAINS AND FLOURS

		Number of calories				Number of calories
Barley, whole-grain, hulled, raw	¼ cup, rounded (makes 1 cup, cooked)	**266**	Oats, rolled, dry, raw	1 cup		**312**
			Potato flour, whole	1 cup		**646**
Buckwheat, whole-grain	⅓ cup, rounded (makes 1 cup, cooked)	**218**	Rice, brown, long-grain (cooked)	1 cup		**232**
			Rice, parboiled (converted, cooked)	1 cup		**186**
Buckwheat flour, dark	1 cup, sifted	**326**	Rice flour	1 cup, stirred		**432**
			Rye flour, dark	1 cup, unsifted		**419**
Buckwheat flour, light	1 cup, sifted	**340**	Rye flour, light	1 cup, unsifted		**364**
Cornmeal:			Wheat, bulgur, dry (parboiled red wheat)	¾ cup (makes 1 cup, cooked)		**452**
Whole-ground, unbolted, dry form	1 cup	**435**				
Degermed—dry form	1 cup	**500**	Wheat flour:			
			Whole-wheat	1 cup, stirred		**400**
Corn grits (hominy grits, cooked)	1 cup	**125**	Whole-wheat pastry flour	1 cup, stirred		**496**
Millet, whole grain	¼ cup, rounded (makes 1 cup, cooked)	**190**	All-purpose, enriched, white flour	1 cup, stirred		**420**
			Wheat germ	1 tbsp		**25**

MEATS, POULTRY, FISH AND EGGS

MEAT, COOKED, WITHOUT BONE*

Beef:			Oven roast:		
Pot roast, braised, or simmered:			Cut relatively fat, such as rib:		
Lean and fat	3 oz (1 thick or 2 thin slices, 4″ x 2⅛″)	**245**	Lean and fat	3 oz (1 thick or 2 thin slices, 4″ x 2¼″)	**375**
Lean only	3 oz (1 thick or 2 thin slices, 4″ x 2⅛″)	**165**	Lean only	3 oz (1 thick or 2 thin slices, 4″ x 2¼″)	**205**

*See pages 99–103 for a guide to portion sizes.

Calorie chart (continued)

		Number of calories			Number of calories
Cut relatively lean, such as round:			Dried beef, chipped	2 oz (about ⅓ cup)	115
Lean and fat	3 oz (1 thick or 2 thin slices, 4″ x 2¼″)	220	Dried beef, creamed	½ cup	190
Lean only	3 oz (1 thick or 2 thin slices, 4″ x 2¼″)	160	Beef and vegetable stew, canned	½ cup	95
Steak, broiled: Cut relatively fat, such as sirloin:			Beef pot pie, home-prepared, baked	¼ pie, 9″ diam	385
Lean and fat	3 oz (1 piece, 3½″ x 2″ x ¾″)	330	Chili con carne, canned	½ cup	240
Lean only	3 oz (1 piece, 3½″ x 2″ x ¾″)	175	Veal: Cutlet, broiled, meat only	3 oz (1 piece, 3¾″ x 2½″ x ⅜″)	185
Cut relatively lean, such as round:			Roast	3 oz (1 thick or 2 thin slices, 4″ x 2¼″)	230
Lean and fat	3 oz (1 piece, 4″ x 2″ x ½″)	220	Lamb: Loin chop (about 3 chops per lb, as purchased):		
Lean only	3 oz (1 piece, 4″ x 2¼″ x ½″)	160	Lean and fat	3½ oz	355
Hamburger patty:			Lean only	about 2⅓ oz	120
Regular ground beef (cooked)	3 oz patty, 2⅝″ diam, ¾″ thick (about 4 patties per lb of raw meat)	245	Leg, roasted: Lean and fat	3 oz (1 thick or 2 thin slices, 4″ x 2¼″)	235
Lean ground beef (cooked)	3 oz patty, 2⅝″ diam, ¾″ thick (about 4 patties per lb of raw meat)	185	Lean only	3 oz (1 thick or 2 thin slices, 4″ x 2¼″)	160
Corned beef, canned	3 oz (1 piece, 4″ x 2½″ x ½″)	185	Shoulder, roasted: Lean and fat	3 oz (1 thick or 2 thin slices, 4″ x 2¼″)	285
Corned beef hash, canned	3 oz (scant ½ cup)	155	Lean only	3 oz (1 thick or 2 thin slices, 4″ x 2¼″)	175

		Number of calories
Pork:		
Fresh		
Chop (about 3 chops per lb, as purchased):		
Lean and fat	about $2\frac{2}{3}$ oz	**305**
Lean only	2 oz	**150**
Roast, loin		
Lean and fat	3 oz (1 thick or 2 thin slices, $3\frac{1}{2}'' \times 2\frac{1}{2}''$)	**310**
Lean only	3 oz (1 thick or 2 thin slices, $3\frac{1}{2}'' \times 2\frac{1}{2}''$)	**215**
Cured:		
Ham:		
Lean and fat	3 oz (1 thick or 2 thin slices, $3\frac{1}{2}'' \times 2\frac{1}{2}''$)	**245**
Lean only	3 oz (1 thick or 2 thin slices, $3\frac{1}{2}'' \times 2\frac{1}{2}''$)	**160**
Bacon, broiled or fried crisp	2 thin slices (28 slices per lb)	**60**
	2 med slices (20 slices per lb)	**85**
Bacon, Canadian	1 slice, $3\frac{3}{8}''$ diam, $\frac{3}{15}''$ thick	**60**
Sausage and variety and luncheon meats:		
Bologna sausage	2 oz (2 very thin slices, $4\frac{1}{2}''$ diam)	**170**
Braunschweiger	2 oz (2 slices, $3\frac{1}{8}''$ diam)	**180**
Vienna sausage, canned	2 oz ($3\frac{1}{2}$ sausages)	**135**
Pork sausage:		
Link	4 links, 4″ long (4 oz uncooked)	**250**

		Number of calories
Bulk	2 patties, $3\frac{7}{8}'' \times \frac{1}{4}''$ (4 oz, uncooked)	**260**
Liver, beef, fried (includes fat for frying)	3 oz (1 piece, $6\frac{1}{2}'' \times 2\frac{3}{8}'' \times \frac{3}{8}''$)	**195**
Heart, beef, braised, trimmed of fat	3 oz (1 thick piece, $4'' \times 2\frac{1}{2}''$)	**160**
Salami	2 oz (2 slices, $4\frac{1}{2}''$ diam.)	**175**
Tongue, beef, braised	3 oz (1 slice, $3'' \times 2'' \times \frac{3}{8}''$)	**210**
Frankfurter	1 frankfurter, 2 oz (8 per lb)	**170**
Broiled ham (luncheon meat)	2 oz (2 very thin slices, $6\frac{1}{4}'' \times 4''$)	**135**
Spiced ham, canned	2 oz (2 thin slices, $3'' \times 2''$)	**165**

POULTRY, COOKED, WITHOUT BONE

Chicken:		
Broiled (no skin)	3 oz (about $\frac{1}{4}$ of a broiler)	**115**
Fried	$\frac{1}{2}$ breast, $2\frac{4}{5}$ oz, meat only	**160**
	1 thigh, $1\frac{4}{5}$ oz, meat only	**120**
	1 drumstick, $1\frac{1}{3}$ oz, meat only	**90**
Canned	$3\frac{1}{2}$ oz ($\frac{1}{2}$ cup)	**200**
Poultry pie, home-prepared, baked	$\frac{1}{4}$ pie, 9″ diam	**410**

Calorie chart (continued)

		Number of calories
Turkey, roasted:		
Light meat (no skin)	3 oz (1 thick or 2 thin slices, 4¼″ x 2″)	**150**
Dark meat (no skin)	3 oz (1 thick or 2 thin slices, 4¼″ x 2″)	**175**

FISH AND SHELLFISH

		Number of calories
Bluefish, baked with fat	3 oz (1 piece, 3½″ x 2″ x ½″)	**135**
Clams, shelled		
Raw, meat only	3 oz (about 4 med clams)	**65**
Canned, clams and juice	3 oz (scant ½ cup, 3 med clams and juice)	**45**
Crabmeat, canned or cooked	3 oz (½ cup)	**80**
Fish sticks, breaded, cooked, frozen (including breading and fat for frying)	3 oz (3 fish sticks, 4″ x 1″ x ½″)	**150**
Haddock, breaded, fried (including fat for frying)	3 oz (1 fillet, 4″ x 2½″ x ½″)	**140**
Mackerel:		
Broiled with fat	3 oz (1 piece, 4″ x 3″ x ½″)	**200**
Canned	3 oz, solids and liquids (scant ½ cup)	**155**

		Number of calories
Ocean perch, breaded, fried (including fat for frying)	3 oz (1 piece, 4″ x 2½″ x ½″)	**195**
Oysters, raw, meat only	½ cup (6–10 med)	**80**
Salmon:		
Broiled or baked	4 oz (1 steak, 4½″ x 2½″ x ½″)	**205**
Canned (pink)	3 oz, solids and liquids (about ⅗ cup)	**120**
Sardines, canned in oil	3 oz, drained solids (7 med sardines)	**170**
Shrimp, canned, meat only	3 oz (27 med shrimp)	**100**
Tuna, canned in oil	3 oz, drained solids (½ cup)	**170**

EGGS

Fried (including fat for frying)	1 large egg	**100**
Hard or soft cooked, "boiled"	1 large egg	**80**
Scrambled or omelet (including milk and fat for cooking)	1 large egg	**110**
Poached	1 large egg	**80**

MILK AND MILK PRODUCTS

MILK, FLUID

Whole	1 cup (8 oz)	**160**
Skim	1 cup (8 oz)	**90**
Partly skimmed (1% fat)	1 cup (8 oz)	**104**
Partly skimmed (2% fat)	1 cup (8 oz)	**145**
Buttermilk	1 cup (8 oz)	**90**

		Number of calories				Number of calories
Evaporated, undiluted	½ cup	**175**	Cheddar	1 oz		**115**
				1 cu ″		**70**
Condensed, sweetened, undiluted	½ cup	**490**		½ cup grated (2 oz)		**230**
			Cottage, large or small curd:			
CREAM			Creamed	1 cup		**235**
Half-and-half (milk and cream)	1 cup	**325**		2 tbsp (1 oz)		**30**
	1 tbsp	**20**	Low fat (2%)	1 cup		**205**
Light, coffee or table	1 tbsp	**30**		2 tbsp (1 oz)		**25**
Sour	1 tbsp	**25**	Low fat (1%)	1 cup		**165**
Whipped topping (pressurized)	1 tbsp	**10**		2 tbsp (1 oz)		**20**
Whipping (volume about double when whipped):			Uncreamed (less than ½ % fat)	1 cup curd		**125**
				2 tbsp (1 oz)		**15**
Light	1 tbsp	**45**	Cream cheese	1 oz		**105**
Heavy	1 tbsp	**55**		1 cu ″		**60**
Imitation cream products (made with vegetable fat):			Parmesan, grated	1 tbsp		**25**
				1 oz		**130**
Creamers:			Swiss	1 oz		**105**
Powdered	1 tsp	**10**		1 cu ″		**55**
Liquid (frozen)	1 tbsp	**20**	Pasteurized processed:			
Sour dressing (imitation sour cream) made with nonfat dry milk	1 tbsp	**20**	American	1 oz		**105**
				1 cu ″		**65**
			Swiss	1 oz		**100**
				1 cu ″		**65**
Whipped topping:			Pasteurized process cheese food:			
Pressurized	1 tbsp	**10**	American	1 tbsp		**45**
Frozen	1 tbsp	**10**		1 cu ″		**55**
Powdered, made with whole milk	1 tbsp	**10**	Pasteurized process cheese spread:			
			American	1 tbsp		**40**
CHEESE				1 oz		**80**
Natural:						
Blue or	1 oz	**105**				
Roquefort type	1 cu ″	**65**	**MILK BEVERAGES**			
Camembert, packed in 4-oz package with 3 wedges per package	1 wedge	**115**	Chocolate, homemade	1 cup		**240**
			Cocoa, homemade	1 cup		**245**

Calorie chart (continued)

		Number of calories				Number of calories
Chocolate-flavored drink made with skim milk and 2% added butterfat	1 cup	190		Rich (about 16% fat)	1 cup	330
Chocolate-flavored drink made with whole milk	1 cup	215		Ice milk:		
				Hardened	1 cup	200
				Soft-serve	1 cup	265
Malted milk	1 cup	245		**YOGURT**		
Chocolate milk shake	1 12-oz container	430		Plain:		
MILK DESSERTS				From skimmed milk	1 cup	125
Custard, baked	1 cup	305		From whole milk	1 cup	150
Ice cream:				Fruit flavored	1 cup	230-75
Regular (about 10% fat)	1 cup	255		Vanilla, coffee, lemon flavored	1 cup	200

NUTS AND SEEDS

Almonds, shelled:				Pecans, chopped	1 cup	810
Slivered	1 cup	690		Pumpkin and squash kernels, dry, hulled	1 cup	775
Chopped	1 cup	775				
Brazil nuts, shelled	6–8 (1 oz)	185				
Cashews, roasted in oil	1 cup	785		Sunflower seeds, dry, hulled	1 cup	810
Filberts (hazelnuts, chopped)	1 cup	730		Sesame seeds, hulled	2 tbsp	94
Peanuts, dry roasted	1 cup	850		Walnuts, black, chopped	1 cup	785
Peanuts, roasted in oil	1 cup	930		Walnuts, Persian or English, chopped (about 60 halves)	1 cup	780
Peanut butter	1 tbsp	95				

SOUPS

Bean with pork	1 cup	170		Cream of asparagus:		
Beef noodle	1 cup	65		With water	1 cup	65
				With milk	1 cup	145
Bouillon, broth, and consommé	1 cup	30		Cream of chicken:		
Chicken gumbo	1 cup	55		With water	1 cup	95
				With milk	1 cup	180
Chicken noodle	1 cup	60		Green pea	1 cup	132
Chicken with rice	1 cup	50		Corn chowder	1 cup	112
Clam chowder, Manhattan	1 cup	80		Vegetable barley	1 cup	166

VEGETABLES AND FRUITS

VEGETABLES

		Number of calories
Asparagus, cooked or canned	6 med spears or ½ cup cut spears	20
Beans:		
Lima, cooked or canned	½ cup	90
Snap, green, wax, or yellow, cooked or canned	½ cup	15
Beets, cooked or canned	½ cup, diced, sliced, or small whole	30
Beets, greens, cooked	½ cup	15
Broccoli, cooked	½ cup chopped or 3 stalks, 4½"–5" long	25
Brussels sprouts, cooked	½ cup, 4 sprouts, 1¼"–1½" diam	25
Cabbage:		
Raw	½ cup, shredded, chopped, or sliced	10
Coleslaw, with mayonnaise	½ cup	85
Coleslaw, with mayonnaise-type dressing	½ cup	60
Carrots:		
Raw	1 carrot, 7½" long, 1⅛" diam	30
	½ cup, grated	25
Cooked or canned	½ cup	25

		Number of calories
Cauliflower, cooked	½ cup flower buds	15
Celery:		
Raw	3 inner stalks, 5" long	10
Cooked	½ cup, diced	10
Chard, cooked	½ cup	15
Chicory, raw	½ cup, ½" pieces	5
Chives, raw	1 tbsp	**trace**
Collards, cooked	½ cup	25
Corn:		
On cob, cooked	1 ear, 5" long, 1¾" diam	70
Kernels, cooked or canned	½ cup	70
Cream style	½ cup	105
Cress, garden, cooked	½ cup	15
Cucumbers, raw, pared	6 center slices, ⅛" thick	5
Dandelion greens, cooked	½ cup	15
Eggplant, cooked	½ cup, diced	20
Endive, raw	½ cup, small pieces	5
Kale, cooked	½ cup	20
Kohlrabi, cooked	½ cup	20
Lettuce, raw	2 large leaves	5
	½ cup, shredded or chopped	5
	1 wedge, ⅙ of head	10
Mushrooms, canned	½ cup	20

Calorie chart (continued)

		Number of calories				Number of calories
Mustard greens, cooked	½ cup	15		Hash browned	½ cup	175
Okra, cooked	½ cup, pods	35		Mashed:		
	½ cup, sliced	25		Milk added	½ cup	70
Onions:				Milk and butter or margarine added	½ cup	100
Young, green, raw	2 med or 6 small, without tops	15		Made from instant granules with milk and butter or margarine added	½ cup	100
	1 tbsp, chopped	5				
Mature:				Pan fried from raw	½ cup	230
Raw	1 tbsp, chopped	5		Salad:		
Cooked	½ cup	30		Made with salad dressing	½ cup	125
Parsley, raw	1 tbsp, chopped	trace		Made with mayonnaise or French dressing and eggs	½ cup	180
Parsnips, cooked	½ cup, diced	50				
	½ cup, mashed	70		Scalloped without cheese	½ cup	125
Peas, cooked or canned	½ cup	65		Sticks	½ cup, pieces ¾″–2¾″ long	95
Peppers, green:						
Raw	1 ring, ¼″ thick	trace		Pumpkin, canned	½ cup	40
	1 tbsp, chopped	trace		Radishes, raw	5 med	5
Cooked	1 med, 2¾″ long, 2½″ diam	15		Rutabagas, cooked	½ cup, diced or sliced	30
Potatoes:						
Au gratin	½ cup	180		Sauerkraut, canned	½ cup	20
Baked	1 potato, 4¾″ long, 2⅓″ diam	145		Spinach, cooked or canned	½ cup	25
Boiled	1 potato, 2½″ diam	90		Squash:		
	½ cup, diced	55		Summer, cooked	½ cup	15
Chips	10 chips, 1¾″ x 2½″	115		Winter:		
				Baked	½ cup, mashed	65
French fried:				Boiled	½ cup, mashed	45
Cooked in deep fat	10 pieces, 3½″–4″ long	215		Sweet potatoes:		
Frozen, heated, ready-to-serve	10 pieces, 3½″–4″ long	170		Baked in skin	1 potato, 5″ long, 2″ diam	160

		Number of calories
Candied	½ potato, 2½" long	160
Canned	½ cup, mashed	140
Tomatoes:		
Raw	1 tomato, 2⅖" diam	20
Cooked or canned	½ cup	30
Tomato juice, canned	½ cup	25
Tomato juice cocktail, canned	½ cup	25
Turnips:		
Raw	½ cup, cubed or sliced	20
Cooked	½ cup, diced	20
Turnip greens, cooked	½ cup	15
Vegetable juice cocktail	½ cup	20
Watercress, raw	10 sprigs	5

DRY LEGUMES

		Number of calories
Black beans, cooked	1 cup	337
Black-eyed peas, cooked	1 cup	190
Garbanzo beans (chickpeas), cooked	1 cup	338
Great Northern beans, cooked	1 cup	210
Lentils, cooked	1 cup	210
Lima beans, cooked	1 cup	262
Mung beans, cooked	1 cup	355
Mung bean sprouts, raw	1 cup	37
Navy beans, cooked	1 cup	225

		Number of calories
Peas, split, cooked	1 cup	230
Pinto or calico beans, cooked	1 cup	330
Red or kidney beans, cooked	1 cup	218
Soybeans, cooked	1 cup	234
Soybeans, cooked, ground	1 cup	416
Soybeans, roasted	1 cup	390
Soybean, fermented (miso)	1 tbsp	29
Soybean curd (tofu)	2½" x 2¾" x 1" piece	86
Soybean flour—low fat	1 cup, stirred	313
Soybean milk, fully fortified	1 cup	155
Soybean protein, dry	1 oz	90
Soybean sprouts, raw	1 cup	48

FRUITS

		Number of calories
Apples, raw	1 med, 2¾" diam (about ⅓ lb)	80
Apple juice, canned	½ cup	60
Applesauce:		
Sweetened	½ cup	115
Unsweetened	½ cup	50
Apricots:		
Raw	3 (about 12 per lb as purchased)	55
Canned:		
Water pack	½ cup, halves and liquid	45
Heavy syrup pack	½ cup, halves and syrup	110
Dried, cooked, unsweetened	½ cup, fruit and juice	105

Calorie chart (continued)

		Number of calories				Number of calories
Avocados:				Figs:		
California varieties	½ of 10-oz avocado, 3⅛″ diam	190		Raw	3 small, 1½″ diam (about ¼ lb)	95
Florida varieties	½ of 16-oz avocado, 3⅝″ diam	205		Canned, heavy syrup	½ cup	110
				Dried	1 large, 2″ x 1″	60
Bananas, raw	1 banana, 6″–7″ long (about ⅓ lb)	85		Fruit cocktail, canned in heavy syrup	½ cup	95
Berries:				Grapefruit:		
Blackberries, raw	½ cup	40		Raw:		
Blueberries:				White	½ med, 3¾″ diam	45
Fresh, raw	½ cup	45			½ cup sections	40
Frozen, sweetened	½ cup	120		Pink or red	½ med, 3¾″ diam	50
Frozen, unsweetened	½ cup	45		Canned (solids and liquid):		
Raspberries:				Water pack	½ cup	35
Fresh, red, raw	½ cup	35		Syrup pack	½ cup	90
Frozen, red, sweetened	½ cup	120		Grapefruit juice:		
Fresh, black, raw	½ cup	50		Fresh	½ cup	50
Strawberries:				Canned:		
Fresh, raw	½ cup	30		Unsweetened	½ cup	50
Frozen, sweetened	½ cup, sliced	140		Sweetened	½ cup	65
				Frozen concentrate, diluted, ready to serve:		
Cantaloupe, raw	½ melon, 5″ diam	80		Unsweetened	½ cup	50
				Sweetened	½ cup	60
Cherries:				Grapes, raw:		
Sour:				American type (including Concord, Delaware, Niagara, and Scuppernong), slip skin	1 bunch, 3½″ x 3″ (about 3½ oz)	45
Raw, with pits	½ cup	30			½ cup with skins and seeds	35
Canned, water pack, pitted	½ cup	50				
Sweet:						
Raw, with pits	½ cup	40		European type (including Malaga, Muscat, Thompson seedless, and Flame Tokay), adherent skin	½ cup	55
Canned:						
Water pack, with pits	½ cup	65				
Syrup pack, with pits	½ cup	105				
Dates, "fresh" or dried, pitted, cut	½ cup	245				

		Number of calories
Grape juice:		
Bottled	½ cup	**85**
Frozen, diluted with 3 parts water by volume	½ cup	**65**
Honeydew melon, raw	1 wedge, 2″ x 7″ (1/10 of melon)	**50**
Lemon juice, raw or canned	½ cup	**30**
	1 tbsp	**5**
Oranges, raw	1 orange, 2⅝″ diam	**65**
Orange juice:		
Fresh	½ cup	**55**
Canned, unsweetened	½ cup	**60**
Frozen concentrate, diluted, ready-to-serve	½ cup	**55**
Peaches:		
Raw	1 med, 2½″ diam (about ¼ lb)	**40**
	½ cup, sliced	**30**
Canned:		
Water pack	½ cup	**40**
Heavy syrup pack	½ cup	**100**
Dried, cooked, unsweetened	½ cup (5–6 halves and liquid)	**100**
Frozen, sweetened	½ cup	**110**
Pears:		
Raw	1 pear, 3½″ long, 2½″ diam	**100**
Canned:		
Water pack	½ cup	**40**
Heavy syrup pack	½ cup	**95**
Pineapple:		
Raw	½ cup, diced	**40**

		Number of calories
Canned in heavy syrup:		
Crushed, tidbits, or chunks	½ cup	**95**
Sliced	1 large slice or 2 small and 2 tbsp juice	**80**
Pineapple juice, canned, unsweetened	½ cup	**70**
Plums:		
Raw:		
Damson	5 plums, 1″ diam (about 2 oz)	**35**
Japanese	1 plum, 2⅛″ diam (about 2½ oz)	**30**
Canned, syrup pack, with pits	½ cup	**105**
Prunes, dried, cooked:		
Unsweetened	½ cup, fruit and liquid	**125**
Sweetened	½ cup, fruit and liquid	**205**
Prune juice, canned	½ cup	**100**
Raisins, dried	½ cup, packed	**240**
Rhubarb, cooked, sweetened	½ cup	**190**
Tangerine, raw	1 med, 2⅜″ diam (about ¼ lb)	**40**
Tangerine juice, canned:		
Unsweetened	½ cup	**55**
Sweetened	½ cup	**60**
Watermelon, raw	1 wedge, 4″ x 8″ (about 2 lb, including rind)	**110**

Calorie chart (continued)

MISCELLANEOUS

		Number of calories				Number of calories
Bouillon cube	1 cube, ½″	**5**	Relishes and sauces:			
Olives:			Chili sauce, tomato	1 tbsp		**15**
Green	5 small, 3 large, or 2 giant	**15**	Tomato ketchup	1 tbsp		**15**
Ripe	3 small or 2 large	**15**	Gravy	2 tbsp		**35**
Pickles, cucumber:			White sauce, med (1 cup milk, 2 tbsp fat, and 2 tbsp flour)	½ cup		**200**
Dill	1 pickle, 4″ long, 1¾″ diam	**15**	Cheese sauce (med white sauce with 2 tbsp grated cheese per cup)	½ cup		**205**
Sweet	1 pickle, 2½″ long, ¾″ diam	**20**				
Popcorn, popped (with oil and salt added)	1 cup large kernels	**40**				

Part 3

Carbohydrates: heroes or villains

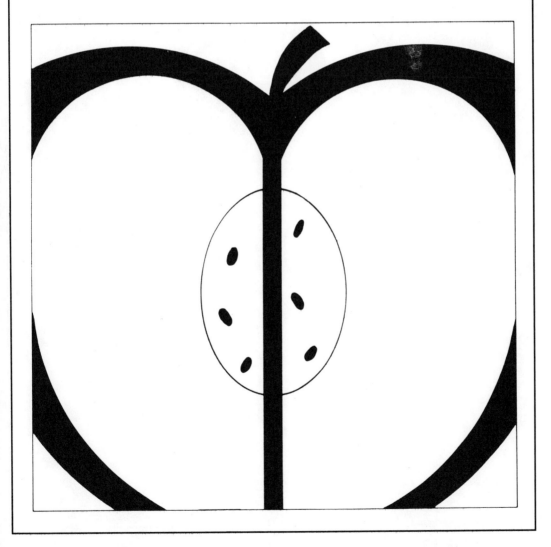

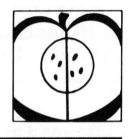

Carbohydrates are often looked upon as the "calorie villains" in our diet. While it is true that carbohydrates are a major source of energy, they can and should provide more than just calories. The problem arises when we eat too much of the empty carbohydrates and too little of the nutritious ones.

As food patterns and eating habits have changed during this century, the amounts and types of carbohydrates that make up our diet have also changed. Not only have we greatly reduced the total amount of these foods, but we have also replaced many of the nutritious carbohydrates (whole grains, fruits, and vegetables) with highly refined flour and sugars. Although the total carbohydrate consumption has dropped by 20 percent since 1910, refined sugars and sweeteners have increased by 35 percent. It now appears that these changes are not without medical consequences. Already they have been linked with several major health problems such as obesity, diabetes, heart disease, and cancer of the colon.

Before reading on, take the following "Self-Assessment." The answers to these questions will begin to get you thinking about carbohydrates and put you in touch with your personal eating habits. After reading the chapter, return to the "Self-Assessment" and take note of your problem areas.

Self-assessment for carbohydrates

☐ Refined sugars

If you consume too much refined sugar, your diet may be high in calories and low in vitamins and minerals. Consider the foods you usually eat and answer the following questions. Record all statements to which you answer "no" in your notebook under the heading "Carbohydrates." Follow the sample on page 172. This record will serve as your personalized plan for improving your diet.

DO YOU USUALLY:

	YES	NO
■ Drink water, club soda, or other no-calorie beverages instead of colas and other sweet sodas?	____	____
■ Drink fruit *juices* rather than fruit *drinks* (for example, orange juice instead of orange drink)?	____	____
■ Drink tea or coffee without sugar?	____	____
■ Have only an occasional serving (twice a week or less) of sweet desserts such as cakes, cookies, pies, or ice cream?	____	____
■ Eat cereals without sugar coating?	____	____
■ Read labels and choose cereals that are low in sucrose and other sugars? (*Low* is equal to less than 5 grams or about 1 teaspoon per serving.)	____	____
■ Read labels to choose foods with the least amount of sugar or other sweeteners?	____	____
■ Eat fresh or water-packed fruits rather than syrup-packed fruits?	____	____
■ Choose whole-grain breads and rolls rather than doughnuts, sweet muffins, or sweet pastries?	____	____
■ Have only an occasional serving (once a week) of candy, or none at all?	____	____

☐ Complex carbohydrates

Eating "whole food" or complex carbohydrates helps to assure that essential minerals, vitamins, and fiber are included in your diet. Answer the following questions to see if you are getting these important foods. Again, record all "no" answers in your notebook.

DO YOU USUALLY:

	YES	NO
■ Eat whole-grain breads and rolls rather than white-flour breads?	_____	_____
■ Choose whole-grain or bran breakfast cereals rather than refined, sugar-coated cereals?	_____	_____
■ Eat at least two servings of raw or lightly steamed vegetables per day?	_____	_____
■ Avoid overcooking vegetables?	_____	_____
■ Eat whole fruits more often than fruit juice (for example, a whole orange versus orange juice)?	_____	_____
■ Eat at least two servings of fruit each day?	_____	_____
■ Choose baked products made from whole-grain (whole wheat, rye, etc.) flour rather than white flour?	_____	_____
■ Have at least four servings of bread or cereals each day?	_____	_____
■ Bake with whole-grain flour rather than white flour?	_____	_____
■ Eat meatless, vegetarian meals with whole grains, legumes, or beans several times a week?	_____	_____
■ Use brown rice instead of white rice?	_____	_____

Self-assessment for carbohydrates (continued)

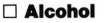

☐ Alcohol

Alcoholic beverages contribute extra calories and little in the way of other nutrients. Remember that calories and sugar are added if the alcohol is combined with a sweet mixer such as tonic, ginger ale, or cola. Consider your alcohol intake by answering the following questions. Record all statements to which you answered "no" in your notebook.

DO YOU USUALLY:

	YES	NO
■ Have an average of not more than one drink a day (one serving equals one jigger of liquor *or* 4 ounces of wine *or* 12 ounces of beer)?	____	____
■ Have wine more often than hard liquor?	____	____
■ Have drinks on the rocks or with noncaloric mixers such as club soda or water?	____	____

Facts to consider

REFINED CARBOHYDRATES

- Sugar has become the predominant source of carbohydrate in our diet, replacing starch or complex carbohydrates.

- A diet high in sugar is often associated with:

  A diet low in fiber or bulk.

  An inadequate intake of vitamins and minerals.

  An increased risk of becoming obese.

  An increased risk of tooth decay (especially if the food is a *sticky* sweet).

- *Refined* carbohydrates are stripped of natural fiber, vitamins, and minerals and are mostly just a source of calories.

- Refined sugar may increase the body's requirements for certain vitamins and minerals while contributing nothing to the diet but calories.

- Refined sugar is rapidly absorbed and requires the body to produce more insulin.

- Although other sweeteners such as honey or brown sugar contain small amounts of nutrients, they are still primarily a concentrated form of calories.

- Much of the sugar in our diet is in beverages. In fact, soft drink consumption has doubled since 1960.

- Be aware of all the various forms of sugar or sweeteners that creep into our diets:

  All those ending in "ose" such as sucrose, glucose, lactose, fructose, and maltose.

  Corn syrup.

  Honey.

  Molasses.

  Maple syrup.

- Sugar is the leading food additive in the United States today.

Facts to consider

COMPLEX CARBOHYDRATES

- *Unrefined* or *whole* fruits, vegetables, and grains are important for supplying fiber, carbohydrate, vitamins, minerals, and calories.

- Enrichment of refined carbohydrates restores only a few of the vitamins and minerals lost in the refining process.

- The American diet has become very high in refined carbohydrate and, therefore, very low in dietary fiber.

- Low-fiber diets have been associated with constipation, diverticulitis, cancer of the colon, appendicitis, hemorrhoids, and hiatus hernia.

- Dietary fiber tends to hold water and produces stools that are bulkier, softer, and pass more quickly and easily through the intestines.

- By creating a softer, bulkier stool, dietary fiber helps to prevent constipation and straining.

- A sudden, large increase in dietary fiber may cause uncomfortable flatulence, cramping, and distention. Add fiber *gradually* to your diet.

- Drink plenty of liquids, especially with more fiber in your diet. Liquids help to avoid gas, constipation, and intestinal blockage.

- The best way to increase dietary fiber is to increase unrefined, high-fiber foods such as whole grains, whole fruits, and vegetables.

- Whole grains spoil and turn rancid more quickly than refined grains. Store tightly sealed in a cool place.

Kernel of Wheat

Aleurone Layers—
Located directly under the bran, these layers contain proteins and the mineral phosphorus.

Bran—
These brown outer layers contain bulk-forming carbohydrates, B-vitamins, and minerals, especially iron.

Endosperm—
This white center is mostly carbohydrate and protein. Only this portion remains in highly refined flours. Partially refined flours and cereals contain endosperm and varying amounts of the aleurone layers.

Germ—
Although only 2¼ percent of the whole kernel, the germ is the heart of the wheat. This embryonic or sprouting section contains thiamin and other B-vitamins, protein, fat, vitamin E, minerals, and carbohydrates.

☐ About carbohydrates

Much of the confusion about the virtues or evils of carbohydrate foods has come from our thinking of them as all being equal. Large variations exist in the nutritional values of different carbohydrate foods.

Carbohydrates in general are the primary source of heat and energy in the body. This energy source is supplied from the starches and sugars in our diet. The term carbohydrate derives from its chemical structure of carbon, hydrogen, and oxygen, with the hydrogen and oxygen present in the same 2-to-1 proportion as in water—hence carbo-hydrate.

Consider the different types of carbohydrates and what they contribute to your diet.

COMPLEX CARBOHYDRATES OR STARCHES

Complex carbohydrates are found as starch in vegetables, grains, and legumes. Starch is the storage form of carbohydrates in plants. It is composed of long chains of sugar molecules (glucose). Because these chains must be broken down to simple sugars before being absorbed by the body, starches supply calories to the bloodstream more slowly than sugar.

Complex carbohydrate foods are important for providing vitamins, minerals, and fiber as well as calories.

SIMPLE CARBOHYDRATES OR SUGARS

Simple carbohydrates are found naturally as part of fruits, vegetables, milk and honey, or as a refined product found in foods such as table sugar, syrups, sodas, cakes, and candy. Simple carbohydrates are more readily absorbed into the body than complex carbohydrates and cause a more rapid increase in blood sugar. *Refined* sugars provide mostly calories and are not of much nutritional value.

FIBER

Fiber is found in whole grains, vegetables, legumes, nuts, and fruits. It is primarily an indigestible form of carbohydrate often referred to as "bulk" or "roughage." It is the portion of the plant cell that provides structure and stability to the plant. There are various types of fiber, including cellulose, hemicellulose, pectins, gums, mucilages, and lignins. Plants differ in the types of fiber they contain. For instance, bran from grain kernels is almost entirely cellulose, while certain fruits such as apples or grapes are high in pectins.

Although much of the fiber in foods is not absorbed by the body, it is considered an important part of the diet. Fiber has a laxative effect, resulting in softer, bulkier stools and a more rapid movement of wastes through the intestinal tract. The various types of fibers such as pectins, cellulose, and lignins seem to contribute a variety of laxative actions, and, therefore, it is important to get a mixture of fibers in the diet.

ALCOHOL

Although not a true carbohydrate, alcohol is derived from carbohydrate foods either by natural fermentation as in wines and beer, or from a distillation process to produce hard liquor such as whisky. Alcoholic beverages, especially those that are distilled, are generally a source of empty calories.

REFINED CARBOHYDRATES

The process of refining carbohydrates tends to strip food of its nutrients, removing essential vitamins, minerals, and fiber. Such processing often results in foods that are high in calories and low in or devoid of everything else.

In refining carbohydrates, the carbohydrate is separated from the original whole-food source. Various refining procedures include removing the bran and wheat germ of grains to make refined flour, polishing rice to make white rice, extracting sugars from fruits and vegetables. For example, whole wheat is refined to make white flour, beets to make sugar, and barley to make alcohol.

WHOLE FOODS

Whole foods is a term used to describe foods in which the carbohydrates and other nutrients have been left intact or have not been separated from the original plant. For example, fruits can be eaten as the original whole fruit, grains can be left as whole grains, or vegetables can be left whole when they are eaten raw or cooked minimally.

Carbohydrates in the "whole" form are a blend of complex, simple, and fibrous forms and retain natural vitamins, minerals, and fibers of the original plant.

☐ **Making changes**

Now that you have taken the "Self-Assessment" and have a better understanding of the variety of carbohydrates, you can see that a number of pros and cons surround the subject of carbohydrates in our diet. Basically, however, making your diet balanced in carbohydrates is rather simple. Keep the following in mind:

- Increase complex carbohydrates.
- Increase fiber.
- Reduce sugar and other refined carbohydrates.

INCREASE COMPLEX CARBOHYDRATES

By increasing the amount of unrefined, whole-food carbohydrates in your diet, you will also be increasing your intake of vitamins, minerals, and fiber. In addition, you will experience the added pleasure of wonderful tastes and textures in your food.

BUY WHOLE-GRAIN BREADS AND CRACKERS

One easy way to increase complex carbohydrates in your diet is to eat whole-grain breads, crackers, and other products baked with whole-grain flours.

Get into the habit of reading labels for the types of flour used in breads you buy. (Remember, you can't always tell from the name.) Ingredients are listed in descending order by weight. The first item listed is the most predominant, and the others follow in descending order.

Consider these two labels for whole grain breads.

The only flour used in the top label is stone-ground whole-wheat. This is the wheat flour highest in fiber. The whole-wheat flour was listed first and therefore is the primary ingredient. In other words, this is a bread high in whole grain.

100% Whole-Wheat Bread
Ingredients: *100% stone-ground whole-wheat flour,* water, corn syrup, partially hydrogenated soybean oil, unsulphured molasses, fresh yeast, salt, nonfat milk, mono- and diglycerides, calcium propionate added to retard spoilage.

Wheat Bread
Ingredients: *Unbleached wheat flour,* cracked wheat, water, *100% stone-ground wheat flour,* corn syrup, unsulphured molasses, partially hydrogenated vegetable shortening, yeast, wheat gluten, salt, honey, vinegar, and mono- and diglycerides (from hydrogenated vegetable oil).

The second label is somewhat more confusing because it reads "Wheat Bread"; one might assume that this is 100% whole-wheat bread. Watch out for this advertising trick. As you can see, the first ingredient is unbleached wheat flour. Although unbleached, this flour is, nevertheless, a *refined* flour in which the bran has been removed. The 100% stone-ground flour is not mentioned until the fourth ingredient, which means it is present in a smaller amount.

Although this bread is white and is more obviously made from refined flour, a look at the ingredients is still interesting. The leading ingredient and source of grain is enriched flour, which is a *refined* wheat flour and probably bleached. Here again all of the fiber of the original whole wheat has been removed along with the

Enriched Bread
Ingredients: *Enriched flour,* water, corn syrup, yeast, partially hydrogenated vegetable shortening, salt, soy flour, calcium sulfate, wheat gluten, sodium stearoyl-2, lactylate, mono- and diglycerides, whey, potassium bromate, calcium propionate.

wheat germ that contains vitamins and minerals. Enrichment replaces some but certainly not all of these nutrients. (See page 58.) Not only is this bread devoid of fiber but it also contains more food additives.

As you can see, choosing a high-fiber bread is tricky business. Take the time to read labels and choose a whole-grain bread.

Of course, you can always make your own whole-wheat bread that will not only be high in fiber but also low in additives. Many specialty and health food stores also carry breads without additives. Remember, however, that without the preservatives breads spoil more quickly. Store whole-grain breads in the refrigerator.

BAKE WITH WHOLE-GRAIN FLOURS
In addition to buying whole-grain breads, get in the habit of using whole-grain flour for cooking and baking. We often hear the argument that white flour is as nutritious as whole-grain flour because it is enriched with B vitamins and iron. What often goes unsaid is that refining flour causes many other losses. Not only are other vitamins and minerals lost through processing, but fiber is also refined away entirely.

Take a look at the chart on the next page to get a view of the extent of nutrient loss when whole-wheat flour is refined.

EAT WHOLE-GRAIN BREAKFAST CEREALS
Many whole-grain cereals are now available, including products made from wheat, oats, rice, and corn. They are not only lower in calories than refined cereals but also rich in vitamins, minerals, and fiber. Read labels carefully. Also, see "Sugar in Cereal" table, page 62.

EAT WHOLE FRUITS
Include whole fruits in your diet more often than fruit juice. For example, for breakfast, eat half a grapefruit instead of drinking grapefruit juice. You will be getting more fiber and more satiety value for your calories.

EAT RAW OR MINIMALLY COOKED VEGETABLES
Raw vegetables provide fiber and are richer in nutrients than cooked ones. If you do cook your vegetables, steam them. Steaming preserves nutrients and some fiber.

Nutrient losses in refining whole wheat to white flour

	Percent loss in white flour	Losses replaced by enrichment
Bran	100	no
Thiamin (Vitamin B_1)	77	yes
Riboflavin (Vitamin B_2)	80	yes
Niacin	81	yes
Vitamin B_6	72	no
Pantothenic Acid	50	no
Folacin	67	no
Alpha-Tocopherol (Vitamin E)	86	no
Choline	30	no
Calcium	60	no
Phosphorus	71	no
Magnesium	85	no
Potassium	77	no
Sodium	78	no
Chromium	40	no
Manganese	86	no
Iron	76	yes
Cobalt	89	no
Copper	68	no
Zinc	78	no
Selenium	16	no
Molybdenum	48	no

Adapted from: Henry A. Schroeder, M.D., "Losses of Vitamins and Trace Minerals Resulting from Processing and Preservation of Food," *The American Journal of Clinical Nutrition* 24 (May 1971):566–69.

INCREASING FIBER

To establish a diet with what is considered to be adequate fiber content, include eight servings *each day* of foods high in fiber. These foods can include whole-grain breads and cereals, whole fruits, and raw or lightly steamed vegetables. While no official recommendation for fiber has been established, eight servings is generally considered a good level. A combination of these foods will help to provide a mixture of different dietary fibers.

If your diet has been low in fiber, add these foods *gradually* to avoid uncomfortable flatulence and distention. Do not overeat fiber. Too much can interfere with absorption of food. Remember to drink plenty of liquid.

TO INCREASE FIBER:

HAVE	INSTEAD OF
Whole-grain breads, rolls, and baked goods	Refined white breads

Breakfast cereals that are whole-grain or bran cereals such as:
    Shredded Wheat
    Wheatena
    Oatmeal
    Grape-Nuts
    All-Bran
	Highly refined cereals with a lot of sugar (i.e., more than 40% of calories from sugar; see table on page 62)

Brown rice	White rice

Whole fruits such as:
    Apples (with skin)
    Bananas
    Peaches (with skin)
    Pears (with skin)
    Plums (with skin) or prunes
    Grapes or raisins
    Strawberries (raw)
	Fruit drinks or fruit juices

More raw vegetables	Cooked, canned, or processed vegetables (these processes break down some of the fiber)
Beans and lentils more frequently	Meats every day

REDUCING SUGAR IN YOUR DIET

Few people realize how much sugar they eat each day—and each year. Even those who are careful about limiting desserts and sweets—the obvious culprits—often take in vast amounts of "hidden" sugar.

Consider the following guidelines for minimizing sugar.

DRINK BEVERAGES THAT
CONTAIN LITTLE OR NO SUGAR

Many people drink a lot of cola and other soft drinks without realizing the amount of sugar and extra calories they contain. Consider the fact that each 12-ounce can of soda contains approximately 150 calories— all from sugar! (There are approximately 15 calories per level teaspoon of sugar.) In fact, drinking soda is probably worse than eating pure sugar because sodas often contain food coloring, caffeine, and other additives as well as empty calories. Consider some alternatives:

Have	Instead of	Sugar Saved (in teaspoons)	Calories Saved
Club soda with a twist of lemon or lime	Colas or other sweet sodas	10 tsp per 12 oz	150 per 12 oz
Fruit juices mixed half and half with club soda	Fruit drinks or pure fruit juice	3–4 tsp per 4 oz	45–60 per 4 oz
Unsweetened tea or coffee*	Tea or coffee with sugar	Varies—$^1/_2$–4+ tsp per cup	8–60+ per cup

*Because of the caffeine in tea and coffee, limit these beverages to no more than four servings per day.

Making such changes can greatly reduce the amount of sugar and calories in your diet, especially for those who tend to drink several sweet sodas or cups of tea and coffee a day. For example, in one year you can save 7,300 teaspoons of sugar or 109,500 calories by eliminating two 12-ounce cans of soda a day. That many extra calories would mean 31 pounds of fat!

REDUCE YOUR INTAKE OF
PROCESSED FOODS

Approximately 70 percent of the sugar we eat is *hidden* in processed foods. It is used not only in soft drinks, sweet desserts, and baked goods but also in many salad dressings, canned and dehydrated soups, pot pies, TV dinners, bacon and other cured meats, some canned and frozen vegetables, all fruit drinks, most canned and frozen fruits, fruit and flavored yogurts, breakfast cereals, ketchup, and other products.

Several suggestions can be made to help minimize sugar in your diet from such products. The most obvious is to minimize the amount of processed foods you use. But since most of us do eat at least some of these foods, the next best thing is to become a label reader.

Try to select products that have the least amount of sugar. Since ingredients are listed in the order of amount by weight, there is at least some basis for comparison. The first item listed is the most predominant, with other ingredients listed in descending order. Be on the lookout not only for sugar but other caloric sweeteners such as dextrose (corn sugar), corn syrup, honey, molasses, and anything ending in *ose*—such as sucrose, glucose, lactose, fructose, or maltose. They are all forms of sugar. The label below from a commercially prepared cake illustrates the various sources of sugar.

In this case, not only is the *first* ingredient sugar, meaning there is more sugar than any other item, but also the fourth and fifth ingredients are sugars in the form of corn syrup and dextrose (or corn sugar).

> **A Popular Cream-Filled Snack Cake**
> Ingredients: *Sugar*, enriched flour, eggs, *corn syrup*, *dextrose*, skim milk, whey, leavening, salt, starch, corn flour, mono- and diglycerides, sodium caseinate, polysorbate 60, artificial color and flavor; sorbic acid.

Besides all the sugar this product contains, it is made from refined, enriched flour and is therefore low in fiber, high in fat, high in calories, and loaded with food additives. Not a very good food if you are looking for good nutrition.

EAT BREAKFAST CEREALS LOW IN SUGAR

Breakfast cereals vary a great deal in the amount of sugar they contain. Some may have only 1 to 2 grams of sugar per serving while others have as much as 14 to 16 grams.

Many cereal labels, such as the one on the right, list the amount of sucrose or sugar in a serving of cereal. The amount is expressed in grams. It is helpful to know there are about 4 grams in a level teaspoon of sugar.

Carbohydrate information
Values by formulation and analysis

	1 oz. (28.4 g)	with ½ cup whole milk
Starch and related carbohydrates	10 g	10 g
Sucrose and other sugars	**8 g***	14 g
Dietary fiber	4 g	4 g
Total carbohydrates	22 g	28 g
***Approximately 2 teaspoons of sugar**		

Help minimize the sugar in your diet by eating the low-sugar cereals. The table on the next page lists many brands according to sugar content.

Sugar in cereal
PERCENT OF CALORIES FROM SUGAR

LESS THAN 15 PERCENT

	Calories from sugar (Percent)		Calories from sugar (Percent)
Cheerios	4	Rice Chex	7
Corn Chex	7	Rice Krispies	11
Corn Flakes	11	Shredded Wheat	0
Corn Total	11	Special K	11
Grape-Nuts	12	Total	11
Product 19	11	Wheat Chex	7
Puffed Rice	0	Wheaties	11
Puffed Wheat	0		

15 TO 50 PERCENT

All-Bran	28.5	Fruity Pebbles	47
Alphabits	40	Golden Grahams	36
Bran Buds	40	Graham Crackers	33
Bran Chex	18	Honeycomb	40
Buc Wheat	18	Life	18
Cap'n Crunch	44	Lucky Charms	40
Cocoa Krispies	47	100% Natural Cereal	17
Cookie Crisp	47	100% Natural Cereal with Brown Sugar & Honey	17
Country Morning	21.5		
Cracklin' Bran	27	100% Natural Cereal with Raisins & Dates	28
Crazy Cow	43		
C. W. Post	22	Quisp	40
Fortified Oat Flakes	24	Raisin Bran	40
40% Bran Flakes	40	Sugar Corn Pops	47
Frosted Flakes	47	Team	18
Frosted Mini Wheats	25	Trix	36
Fruit Loops	47		

GREATER THAN 50 PERCENT

Apple Jacks	55
Sugar Smacks	58
Super Sugar Crisp	51

In choosing a breakfast cereal also try to minimize food colorings, additives, and refined grains.

For example, consider the following two sample cereals.

Cereal #1
Ingredients: 100% natural whole wheat; BHT, a preservative, is added to the packaging to retain the natural whole-wheat flavor.

Cereal #2
Ingredients: Sugar, corn, wheat and oat flour, salt, corn syrup, dried apples, cinnamon, partially hydrogenated vegetable oil (one or more of coconut, soybean, and palm), sodium ascorbate (C), natural apple flavoring, vitamin A, palmitate, artificial coloring, niacinamide, ascorbic acid (C), baking soda, reduced iron, zinc oxide, thiamin hydrochloride (B_1), pyridoxine hydrochloride (B_6), riboflavin (B_2), folic acid, and vitamin D. BHA added to preserve product freshness.

Cereal #1 is by far a better choice—it is a whole-grain cereal, with no sugar or additives. The preservative is in the packaging and not the cereal itself.

In contrast, Cereal #2 is loaded with sugar, made from refined flour, and contains hydrogenated fat, colorings, and other additives.

All things considered, here are some of the better cereals available:

- Familia
- Grape-Nuts
- Maltex*
- Oatmeal* (long cooking type)
- Ralston*
- Rice and Wheat Chex
- Shredded Wheat

---

*Hot cereals often contain more whole grains and less sugar than cold cereals, but here again check the food label.

EAT FRESH FRUITS

To help cut down on sugar, try to eat primarily fresh fruits. Try to avoid canned fruits, but if you do eat them, drain or rinse the syrup from them. The syrup is primarily sugar.

CUT DOWN ON SWEET DESSERTS

Obviously the best way to avoid the sugar in desserts is to eliminate sweet desserts altogether. It isn't necessary to go that far, but consider the number of desserts you eat each week and think about cutting out some of them. Also, substitute fresh fruit for high-sugar, high-calorie desserts (cake, pudding, pie). Remember too, that many desserts that are high in sugar are also high in fat. Below is a list of common desserts together with the number of teaspoons of sugar in one serving:

	SERVING SIZE	TEASPOONS OF SUGAR
Iced layer cake*	$1/12$ cake	9
Cheese cake*	$1/12$ cake	4
Ice cream*	$1/2$ cup	4
Italian ice	$1/2$ cup	8
Gelatin desert	$1/2$ cup	4
Apple pie*	$1/6$ pie	5 $1/3$
Butterscotch pudding*	$1/2$ cup	10
Tapioca pudding*	$1/2$ cup	6
Sherbet	$1/2$ cup	5 $1/3$

*Also high in fat.

AVOID OR LIMIT CANDY

Many candies are made up almost entirely of sugar. One-half cup of jelly beans has the equivalent of 27 teaspoons of sugar! Like many desserts, candy such as fudge and chocolate are not only high in sugar, but also high in fat. Keep candy consumption to a minimum.

EAT PLAIN YOGURT

Yogurt is often categorized as a "health food," but the fact is that many commercial yogurts are high in sugar. Vanilla, coffee, and fruit yogurts are usually highly sugared—vanilla, coffee, and lemon yogurt having an equivalent of $3\frac{1}{2}$ teaspoons of sugar per 8 ounces and fruit yogurts having up to 7 teaspoons.

If you enjoy yogurt, try buying plain yogurt and adding fresh fruit. You will eliminate the excess sugar and will probably have a better tasting yogurt.

Sugar in foods

The following list shows the approximate amount of refined sugar in teaspoons per serving.

Food	Serving size	Tsp of sugar
Bran muffin (homemade)	1 muffin (2″)	$\frac{1}{3}$
Iced layer cake	1 piece ($\frac{1}{12}$ cake)	9
Cereal—sugar coated	1 cup	5
Cheese cake	$\frac{1}{12}$ cake	4
Coffee cake	1 piece, 3″ x 3″	$4\frac{1}{3}$
Chocolate fudge	1 piece, 1″ x 1″	$2\frac{1}{4}$
Hard candy	1 oz	7
Vanilla ice cream	$\frac{1}{2}$ cup	4
Italian ice	$\frac{1}{2}$ cup	8
Jam	1 tbsp	3
Gelatin dessert	$\frac{1}{2}$ cup	4
Ketchup	$\frac{1}{4}$ cup	$\frac{1}{2}$
Apple pie	$\frac{1}{6}$ pie	$5\frac{1}{3}$
Butterscotch pudding	$\frac{1}{2}$ cup	10
Tapioca pudding	$\frac{1}{2}$ cup	6
Lime sherbet	$\frac{1}{2}$ cup	$5\frac{1}{3}$
Soda—cola or other sweet sodas	12 oz can	10
Vanilla or coffee yogurt	1 cup (8 oz)	$3\frac{1}{2}$
Fruit yogurt	1 cup (8 oz)	7

Getting the most from carbohydrate foods does take some thought, but as you can see, there are many choices. Remember, it is the whole-food carbohydrates—fruits, vegetables, whole grains—that provide more than just sugar and extra calories.

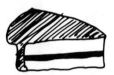

1 piece cake

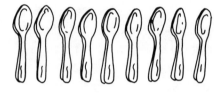

9 tsp sugar

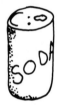

12 oz can soda

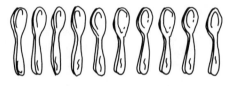

10 tsp sugar

1 cup sugar-coated cereal

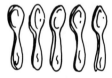

5 tsp sugar

1 tbsp jam

3 tsp sugar

½ cup Italian ice

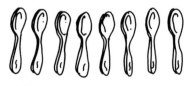

8 tsp sugar

Part 4

Fat: the controversial nutrient

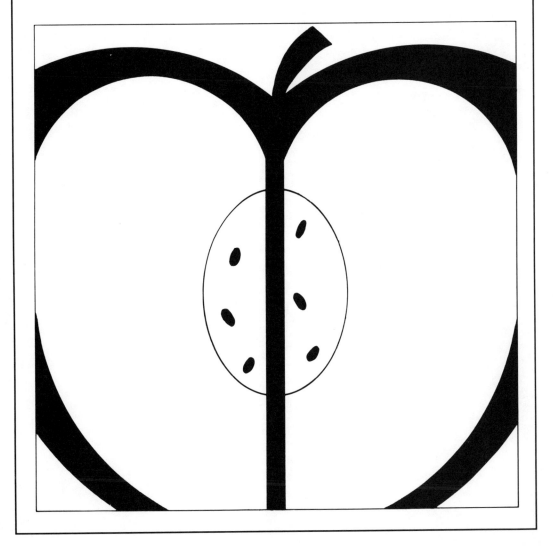

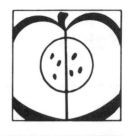

The increase in fat consumption is one of the most obvious and potentially dangerous changes in modern dietary patterns. It has been estimated that fat provides 42 percent of our calories. This represents an increase of 31 percent over the diet of Americans in 1910. Although there is still some controversy concerning what to do about fat in the diet, it now appears advisable for us to lower fat consumption to 30 to 35 percent of our calories.

Why has fat consumption increased? One important factor, which may surprise you, is the significant increase in "separated" fats (fats extracted from their natural source) such as margarine, vegetable oils, and shortening. Although these fats are of vegetable origin and, therefore, generally low in saturated fat and cholesterol, we are eating too much of them. We must not only monitor the *kind* of fat in our diet, but the *total amount* of fat as well.

Consumption of fats derived from meats has also increased, so that nearly one-third of the fat in our diet comes from red meats alone. This increase has partially offset the decrease in saturated fats from butter and lard.

One of the primary concerns about dietary fat arises from the fact that it is a "calorie-loaded" nutrient. Fats contain more than *twice* the amount of calories per gram as protein and carbohydrates. More important, fatty foods tend to have a low amount of vitamins and minerals relative to their caloric content. Unfortunately, fatty foods have been replacing many of the nutritious whole grains and fresh fruits and vegetables that used to be prevalent in the American diet. Consequently, we have been reducing not only the variety of tastes and textures provided by nutritious foods but also the valuable vitamins, minerals, and fiber they can provide (see Part 3, "Carbohydrates"). To put it succinctly, we have been trading low-calorie, high-nutrient foods for calorie-packed, low-nutrient fats.

As the amount of fat in our diet has changed, so have the patterns of chronic health problems. The high-fat diet has been correlated with such serious problems as obesity, heart disease, and cancer of the colon, breast, and prostate. Although there is still some uncertainty as to the precise relationship of fat to disease, it would seem wise for us to play it safe by eating less fat.

Self-assessment for fat

Evaluate your diet for both the total fat content and the type of fat you are eating. Consider each of the following questions and record all statements to which you answer "no" in your notebook. Follow the sample on page 172.

☐ Total fat

DO YOU:

	YES	NO
■ Have fish and poultry more frequently than red meats?	____	____
■ Have meatless meals (without red meat, fish, or chicken) at least two full days a week?	____	____
■ Have an average meat intake of no more than 21 to 28 ounces per week, or 3 to 4 ounces a day?	____	____
■ Have no more than one serving a week or none at all of high-fat luncheon meats (franks, bologna, salami, liverwurst, etc.)?	____	____
■ Select lean cuts of meat (little visible fat)?	____	____
■ Broil or roast rather than fry meats?	____	____
■ Trim any visible fat from meats?	____	____
■ Have no more than 4 ounces of cheese a week (other than cottage cheese)?	____	____
■ Use salad dressings sparingly (1 tablespoon per serving) or not at all?	____	____
■ Choose low-fat snacks (such as raw vegetables, fruits, whole-grain crackers, or plain yogurt) rather than nuts and chips?	____	____
■ Use butter, margarine, and mayonnaise sparingly or not at all on breads, rolls, and vegetables?	____	____
■ Have fruit for dessert rather than cakes, cookies or pies?	____	____
■ Have vegetables that are steamed, boiled, or baked rather than french fried or pan fried?	____	____

☐ **Saturated fat and cholesterol**

DO YOU USUALLY:

	YES	NO
■ Limit egg yolks to 3 to 4 a week?	____	____
■ Have not more than four servings of red meat a week (beef, lamb, pork)?	____	____
■ Have skim milk or low-fat buttermilk rather than whole milk?	____	____
■ Avoid eating the visible fat on meats?	____	____
■ Have liver not more than once a week?	____	____
■ Have only an occasional serving of sour cream and sour cream dips and dressings?	____	____
■ Use butter sparingly or not at all?	____	____
■ Have cheeses made from skimmed milk or partially skimmed milk rather than from cream or whole milk?	____	____
■ Have broth soups rather than creamed soups?	____	____
■ Skim the fat off stews and soups?	____	____
■ Skim the fat off meat juices before making gravy?	____	____
■ Have no more than an occasional serving of commercial cakes, pies, or cookies?	____	____
■ Use milk (preferably skim) in tea or coffee rather than cream or creamers (powder or liquid)?	____	____
■ Have only an occasional serving of ice cream?	____	____

Facts to consider

■ Although some fat is necessary in the diet, fats are essentially "empty calories" providing very little in the way of vitamins and minerals.

■ Because people today are generally less active than they used to be, fewer calories are required in the diet. Be careful not to "waste" calories with too many fats.

■ It is generally recommended that fats be limited to 30 to 35 percent of total calories.

■ Much of the fat in our diet is in "protein" foods such as meat, cheese, eggs, milk, and nuts. Some of the popular "protein" foods are very high in fat; most hamburgers have approximately 65 percent of the calories as fat, most cheeses contain 70 percent fat calories, and many nuts 70 percent fat calories.

■ Nearly half the fat in chicken is in the skin.

■ Eating fish can help to keep fat intake low; fish is generally much lower in fat than red meats and poultry.

■ Use only small amounts of salad dressings, oils, and mayonnaise, and use margarine or butter sparingly, to reduce the fats in your diet.

■ Diets high in saturated fat and cholesterol tend to elevate blood cholesterol and triglyceride levels. High blood fats have been linked with increased risk of heart disease. However, individuals vary in their susceptibility toward elevated blood fats. It is wise to know your levels.

■ Saturated fats are mostly found in such animal foods as meats, eggs, and cheese. In addition, some vegetable oils such as palm oil and coconut oil contain large amounts of saturated fat. Many processed foods such as bakery products, nondairy creamers, and packaged desserts contain saturated fats in this form.

■ Cholesterol is found only in fats from animals. These include red meats, poultry, eggs, cheese, and shellfish.

■ While dietary cholesterol and saturated fats tend to *increase* blood cholesterol, polyunsaturated fats tend to *decrease* it.

■ The American diet tends to be high in saturated fat and cholesterol. A better balance would be an even distribution of polyunsaturated, monounsaturated, and saturated fats.

Fat in your foods

% Calories from fat

Food	10	30	50	70	90

Cheddar cheese — bar to ~70

Cottage cheese — bar to ~32

Chicken—white meat (without skin) — bar to ~18

Chicken—dark meat (without skin) — bar to ~30

Bologna — bar to ~87

Frankfurter — bar to ~87

Haddock — small bar

Lean beef—flank steak — bar to ~30

Fatty beef—ground beef — bar to ~63

Salad dressing — bar to ~90

Peanuts — bar to ~80

Ice cream — bar to ~48

Peach — small bar

Cookie—chocolate chip — bar to ~33

☐ About fats

Fats, whether in the body or in foods, are chemical compounds made up of carbon, hydrogen, and oxygen. The more scientific name for fats is lipids, but the terms are often used interchangeably. They are important for providing energy, serve as building blocks for hormones, carry fat-soluble vitamins (A,D,E,K), form a protective cushion around vital organs, and make up part of the structure of individual cells.

There are three main types of fats or lipids: triglycerides, cholesterol, and phospholipids. Each has a different structure and different functions, but all of them have the common lipid characteristic of being insoluble in water (or blood). In order for lipids to be carried in the bloodstream, they must be attached to proteins—forming lipoproteins. The lipoproteins transport fats to organs and adipose tissue for cellular use and storage. When there is an excess of lipoproteins carrying cholesterol, the cholesterol is more likely to be deposited in the blood vessels, which hastens the onset of hardening of the arteries or arteriosclerosis.

MORE ABOUT THE THREE MAIN LIPIDS

TRIGLYCERIDES

Dietary fat and body fat are mostly in the form of triglycerides. It is this form of lipid that is commonly called fat. The grams of fat in oil, butter, margarine, meats, dairy products, and other foods are triglycerides, as are fats stored in the body. The term triglyceride refers to the chemical structure that consists of three *fatty acids* (tri) linked to a glycerol (glyceride) molecule as shown in the illustration below.

Chemical structure for a triglyceride

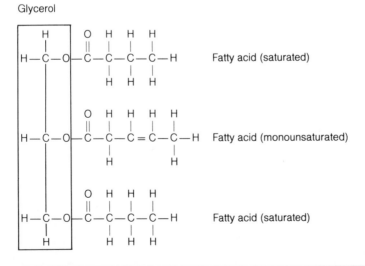

Glycerol

Fatty acid (saturated)

Fatty acid (monounsaturated)

Fatty acid (saturated)

Fatty acids are composed of carbon atom (C) chains with hydrogen (H) atoms attached along the chain. In addition to the hydrogen, there is an acid group at one end of the chain.

These chains may contain only a few carbons, such as the fatty acids found in dairy products, which have six to ten carbon atoms, or long chains of sixteen or more carbons, which are predominantly in the fats found in meat, fish, and oils.

Linoleic acid

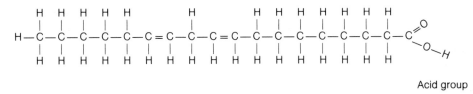

Acid group

The illustration above shows an eighteen-carbon fatty acid called linoleic acid. Linoleic acid is the only fatty acid that must be provided in the diet; therefore, it is called an essential fatty acid. It is found in vegetable oils such as corn or safflower oil. While other fatty acids are important for growth, reproduction, and healthy skin, they can be manufactured in the body. Linoleic acid cannot.

Fats are described as "saturated" or "polyunsaturated" according to the fatty acids that make up the triglyceride molecule. For example, the triglyceride in the illustration on page 74 would be called a saturated fat because two of the three fatty acids are saturated. A closer look at the components of triglycerides will help to distinguish the differences in these fats.

Saturated fats are named for fats in which the triglyceride contains a predominance of saturated fatty acids.

Saturated fatty acid

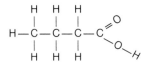

Carbon atoms (C) are saturated or surrounded by hydrogen atoms (H)

This saturation results in a fat that is solid at room temperature. Saturated fats are most often found in animal fats such as meat fat, butter, and certain creams.

Monounsaturated fatty acid

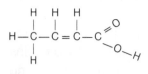

One pair of carbon atoms (C) are unsaturated with hydrogen atoms (H)

With *monounsaturated fats,* the carbon chain has one pair of carbon atoms that are unsaturated (mono) with hydrogen atoms. In the above illustration, the double line between the carbon atoms identifies the unsaturated bond.

Because of the unsaturated carbons, this type of fat is slightly more fluid than saturated fats and is, therefore, liquid at room temperature but still solid when chilling. Avocados, cashews, and olive oil are foods high in monounsaturated fats.

Polyunsaturated fatty acid

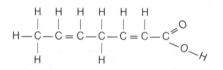

Two or more pairs of carbon atoms (C) are unsaturated

Liquid at room temperature as well as upon chilling, *polyunsaturated fats* are found in vegetable oils such as corn or safflower oil. Polyunsaturated fats are often transformed into saturated fats by a process called hydrogenation. During this process, the polyunsaturated oil is transformed by bubbling hydrogen into it. The unsaturated carbons of the oil are therefore saturated, with hydrogens changing liquid oils to hardened fats.

CHOLESTEROL

Another fatlike substance of importance is cholesterol. Although different in chemical structure from triglycerides, cholesterol is also in the category of fats or lipids. Cholesterol is found in all body tissue, especially the brain, nerves, adrenal cortex, and liver. It is also a component of bile, serves as a precursor for vitamin D, and is involved in the synthesis of some hormones.

Cholesterol in the body comes from two sources: it is supplied in the diet and it is synthesized by the body. The amount of cholesterol synthesized is somewhat dependent on the amount provided by the diet; if you eat more the body produces less. However, it is possible to overload this balance, resulting in elevated blood levels. In fact, the body is capable of making all the cholesterol it requires and does not need a supply from the diet at all.

The three types of fatty acids in the diet tend to affect blood cholesterol levels in different ways. Saturated fats tend to elevate blood cholesterol levels, although the mechanism by which this occurs is not known. Because elevated blood cholesterol is associated with an increased risk for heart disease, it is advisable to limit the amount of saturated fat that is eaten. Monounsaturated fats tend to have little or no effect on blood cholesterol levels. Polyunsaturated fats tend to lower blood cholesterol levels and are, therefore, encouraged as a substitute for saturated fats. Many people confuse this recommended substitution for dietary supplementation, and are under the impression that polyunsaturated fats should be increased in the diet. This is not the case because they also contribute to total fat and have just as many calories as other types of fats.

PHOSPHOLIPIDS

Phospholipids are similar in chemical structure to triglycerides except that one of the three fatty acids is replaced by a phosphorus-containing compound. The most common form of phospholipid in the body is lecithin. It is an important part of the membrane of cells and a component of the covering of nerves. It also plays a role in the coagulation of blood. Lecithin is produced in the liver, and for this reason there is no known dietary deficiency of this substance in man.

HOW LIPIDS ARE CARRIED IN THE BLOOD

In order for lipids to be carried in the blood as soluble material, they must be attached to protein molecules, thus forming lipoproteins. There are different types of lipoproteins carrying varying amounts of cholesterol, triglycerides, and other lipids. Lipoproteins are divided into three types by their density: very low density lipoproteins—VLDL, low density lipoproteins—LDL, and high density lipoproteins—HDL. Cholesterol is found predominantly in the low density and high density lipoproteins, whereas triglycerides are found predominantly in the very low density lipoproteins.

Physicians are now interested in measuring both total blood cholesterol and the HDL:LDL ratio when evaluating a patient's risk factors for heart disease. High levels of HDL in the blood are thought to be a "protective" factor in heart disease, whereas high levels of LDL are linked with increased risk. Much more research is needed, however, before we know conclusively the role that these lipoproteins play in the development of atherosclerosis and heart disease.

HOW LIPIDS ARE STORED IN THE BODY

When there is an excess of lipids beyond the energy needs of the body, the extra fat is stored as adipose tissue, the common yellow-gold fat that we are most familiar with. When our calorie intake is restricted, the body can mobilize this adipose tissue to meet the body's energy needs. The key to reducing the adipose tissue (or body fat) is to lower the *total amount of calories* ingested, not just fat, for if calorie ingestion is high in the form of carbohydrates even though it is low in fat, the body will utilize the carbohydrates as energy sources instead of the adipose tissue. More important, carbohydrates can be converted into fat and stored as adipose tissue.

Foods and their fats

High in polyunsaturated fats	Moderate in polyunsaturated fats	High in monounsaturated fats	High in saturated fats
Safflower oil	Soybean oil	Peanut oil	Meat: Beef, lamb, pork, pork products such as luncheon meats, sausages
Corn oil	Cottonseed oil	Olive oil	
Walnuts	Soft tub margarines	Olives	
Soynuts	Commercial salad dressings (most)	Avocados	Chicken fat
Sunflower seeds	Mayonnaise	Almonds	Meat drippings
Sesame seeds		Pecans	Lard
Products made with the above		Cashews	Hydrogenated shortening
		Peanuts	Coconut oil
		Brazil nuts	Palm oil
			Stick margarines
			Butter
			Whole milk
			Whole milk cheese
			Cream: sweet and sour
			Ice cream
			Ice milk
			Chocolate
			Coconut
			Products made with the above, such as most cakes, pastry, cookies, gravy, nondairy creamers, sauces, and many snack foods

☐ Making changes

Let the following guide help you to be "fat wise" when making food choices. The overall goals are to:

- Reduce total fat.
- Reduce cholesterol.
- Balance the types of fat by having less saturated fat.

THE RIGHT FOOD CHOICE CAN HELP ACHIEVE SEVERAL GOALS AT ONCE

Food choice	Reduce total fat	Reduce cholesterol	Reduce saturated fat	Increase polyunsaturated fat
Eat less meat	■	■	■	
Have lean meats, poultry, fish	■	■	■	
Limit high-fat cheeses	■	■	■	
Limit butter	■	■	■	
Have vegetable oil instead of hydrogenated shortening			■	■
Use skim milk	■	■	■	
Eat 3 eggs or less per week		■		
Avoid or limit rich desserts (cakes, pies, cookies, ice cream)	■	■	■	
Have low-fat snacks	■		■	

EAT LESS MEAT

Americans tend to overeat meat, which is a primary source of both protein and fat. By limiting meat to an average of 3 to 4 ounces a day or 21 to 28 ounces per week, you will get plenty of protein while reducing the amount of animal fat in your diet.

A delightful way to limit meat and still get protein in your diet is to enjoy meatless meals. Use whole grains, legumes, and low-fat milk dishes to help cut down on fats, provide good sources of protein, and make your meals more interesting. (See section on meatless meals, pages 104–05.)

Stretch meat by cutting it up and mixing it with vegetables oriental style or by including it in a casserole.

EAT LEAN MEAT, POULTRY, AND FISH

Eating more fish and poultry than red meat helps to keep fat levels low. Most fish are very low in total fat and saturated fat and therefore are a good choice. But fish do contain some cholesterol, so don't overeat this protein food either. Shrimp, lobster, and crab are higher in cholesterol than other fish; have them less often.

Chicken, turkey, and Cornish hens also are lower in total fat, especially if eaten without the skin. The light meat has less fat than dark meat.

By choosing red meats that are lean and trimmed of visible fat, you can avoid a lot of saturated fat. Remember that even lean meats contain some saturated fat and cholesterol, so limit how much you eat. Choose meats graded as choice rather than prime; they are lower in fat. For suggestions, see the table on the next page.

Meat selection

LOW-FAT MEATS

Fish

Bass	Oysters
Brook trout	Perch
Cod	Swordfish
Crappie (Sunfish)	Water-packed tuna
Flounder	Scallops
Haddock	Lobster*
Clams	Crab*
	Shrimp*

Poultry (without skin)

Chicken	Cornish hen
Turkey	

Veal (trim any visible fat)

Sirloin roast and steak	Loin chop
Arm steak	Rump roast

Beef (trim any visible fat)

Round roast	Smoked beef
Ground round (have	Flank steak
fat removed before	Tenderloin
grinding)	Dried beef
	Corned beef round

Lamb (trim any visible fat)

Roast leg	Loin chop

Pork (trim any visible fat)

Sirloin roast	Tenderloin
Center-cut loin chop	Lean ham
Center-cut ham steak	Canadian bacon

HIGH-FAT MEATS

Highly marbled meats—with visible fat throughout meat

Organ meats—kidney, heart, liver (high in iron and vitamins; they should not be excluded from diet)

Canned meat products

Luncheon meats—salami, bologna, liverwurst, etc.

Hamburger

Frankfurters

Sausages

Spareribs

Pork butts

Picnic shoulder

Pork steak

Bacon

Veal cutlets

Lamb blade chops

Corned beef brisket

All poultry skin

Goose

Duck

*Lobster, shrimp, and crab are very low in total fat but somewhat high in cholesterol.

Table adapted from "A Maximal Approach to the Dietary Treatment of the Hyperlipidemias," Booklet B, American Heart Association Publication, p. 19.

LIMIT HIGH-FAT CHEESES

Although many "health diets" contain a lot of cheese for the protein content, it must be remembered that most cheeses are also very high in total fat, especially saturated fat. Some also contain a considerable amount of cholesterol.

It isn't necessary to avoid cheese, but try to limit the amount of high-fat cheese to 2 to 4 ounces a week. Also, use your cheese in meatless meals, not in addition to meat.

Although no cheese is very low in fat, some are much lower then others. Help keep fat low by selecting the lower-fat cheeses. See the table below.

LOWER-FAT CHEESES	Calories from fat (percent)	HIGH-FAT CHEESES	Calories from fat (percent)
Low-fat cottage cheese	19.3	Feta cheese	72.6
Creamed cottage cheese	39.4	Cream cheese	90.0
Mozzarella—part skim	56.3	Mozzarella—whole milk	69.2
Ricotta—part skim	51.5	Ricotta—whole milk	67.2
Grated parmesan	59.2	Swiss	65.8
		Cheddar	73.9
		American	75.1
		Gruyère	70.4
		Muenster	73.4
		Camembert	72.8
		Brie	74.6

USE BUTTER SPARINGLY

Use butter sparingly or not at all. By doing so, you will reduce the amounts of total fat, saturated fat, and cholesterol.

You may choose to use margarine instead of butter, and this should help to lower saturated fat intake. But go sparingly with margarine also; remember that it has the same amount of fat and calories as butter and that at least some of the polyunsaturated vegetable oil has been hydrogenated. Hydrogenation gives the product more of a hardened, buttery texture, but unfortunately the process changes the natural structure of the vegetable oil and makes it a more saturated fat.

USE POLYUNSATURATED OILS

Use polyunsaturated vegetable oils instead of hydrogenated shortening or saturated oils. In this way the amount of saturated fat will be reduced while the polyunsaturates will increase. Again, use oils sparingly to keep total fat and calories down. The most polyunsaturated oils are derived from safflower, corn, and walnuts. Some of the more saturated oils include coconut oil and palm oil. Read labels to check for these fats.

DRINK SKIM MILK

Drink skim milk or low-fat milk (1%) instead of whole milk or cream. Low-fat milk has less total fat, less saturated fat, and less cholesterol. Be aware of foods made with cream and whole milk. Read labels carefully to check for these ingredients.

EAT FEWER EGGS

Limit eggs to not more than three a week. Eggs are very high in cholesterol, and too many in the diet can elevate blood cholesterol levels. Be certain to count the eggs used in cooking as well as those eaten directly.

MINIMIZE RICH DESSERTS

Cakes, cookies, pies, ice cream, and other rich desserts are often not only high in fats but also high in saturated fat and cholesterol. This is especially true of commercially prepared products. When preparing desserts at home use low-fat milk products and polyunsaturated fats.

EAT LOW-FAT SNACKS

If you are going to snack, save fat and calories by enjoying snacks of fresh fruits, raw vegetables, and plain, low-fat yogurt. Watch out for fatty potato chips, dips, peanut butter, seeds, and nuts. While peanut butter, seeds, and nuts do have protein and other nutrients, they also are very high in fat (at least 70 percent of their calories are derived from fat). One of the better choices is soynuts, which have 40 percent calories from fat.

COOK WITH LESS FAT

Cooking methods can make a difference. Get in the habit of doing the following when preparing foods:

- Trim away all visible fat before cooking meat.
- Broil, roast, and bake rather than fry.
- Use a rack to drain off fat when cooking meats.

- Skim away fat when making soups and stews (by chilling the stock so that the fat hardens on top).

- Cook with polyunsaturated or low-fat ingredients such as polyunsaturated margarines, low-fat cheeses, or skim milk products.

Become "fat wise" in your food choices and preparation. Review your self-assessment and begin to plan changes for minimizing the fat in your diet.

Cholesterol content of food

	Amount	Cholesterol (mg)		Amount	Cholesterol (mg)
EGGS	1 large	**252**	Flounder, flesh only	3 oz, raw	**42**
BEEF			Haddock, flesh only	3 oz, raw	**51**
Lean, trimmed of separable fat	3 oz, cooked	**77**	Halibut, flesh only	3 oz, raw	**42**
Beef brains	1 oz, raw	**560**	Herring, flesh only	3 oz, raw	**72**
CHICKEN			Lobster, meat only	3 oz, cooked	**72**
Breast, meat only	3 oz, cooked	**67**	Mackerel, flesh only	3 oz, raw	**81**
Drumstick, meat only	3 oz, cooked	**77**	Oysters, meat only	3 oz, raw	**42**
FISH			Salmon, sockeye or red	3 oz, raw	**30**
Clams, soft shell	½ dozen (7.2 oz), in shell; approx. 2.5 oz raw meat	**36**	Sardines, canned and drained	3 oz	**117**
Clams, hard shell	4 chowder clams; approx. 4.6 oz raw meat	**65**	Scallops, muscle only	3 oz, raw	**30**
			Shrimp, flesh only	3 oz, raw	**126**
Crab, all kinds Steamed, meat only	¼ cup (1.1 oz)	**31**	Trout, flesh only	3 oz, raw	**45**
Canned	¼ cup (1.4 oz)	**40**	Tuna, canned and drained	3 oz	**54**
			LAMB		
			Lean, trimmed of separable fat	3 oz, raw	**60**

	Amount	Cholesterol (mg)		Amount	Cholesterol (mg)
LIVER			**CHEESE**		
Including beef, calf, hog, and lamb liver	3 oz, raw	**255**	Cream	1 tbsp	**16**
			Cottage, 1% fat	1 cup	**10**
Chicken liver	3 oz, raw	**472**	Cottage, 4% fat	1 cup	**31**
PORK			Cottage, uncreamed	1 cup	**10**
Lean, trimmed of separable fat	3 oz, raw	**51**	Cheddar, mild or sharp	1 oz	**30**
MILK AND CREAM			Mozzarella, low moisture, part skim	1 oz	**15**
Milk, whole	1 cup	**33**	Ricotta, partially skim milk	½ cup	**38**
Milk, low-fat 2%	1 cup	**18**			
Milk, low-fat 1%	1 cup	**10**	**CAKE**		
Milk, skim	1 cup	**4**	Angel food cake	¹⁄₁₂ of 10″ cake	**0**
Buttermilk, cultured from nonfat milk	1 cup	**5**	Devil's food cake	¹⁄₁₆ of 9″ cake	**33**
Half and half (milk and cream)	1 cup	**89**	Sponge cake	¹⁄₁₂ of 10″ cake	**162**
Ice cream, 10% fat (regular)	½ cup	**29**	Dark fruit cake	¹⁄₃₀ of 8″ loaf	**7**
Ice cream, 16% fat (rich)	½ cup	**44**	**FATS**		
Ice milk	½ cup	**7**	Butter	1 tbsp	**31**
Sherbet	½ cup	**7**	Lard	1 tbsp	**12**

Part 5

Protein: too much of a good thing

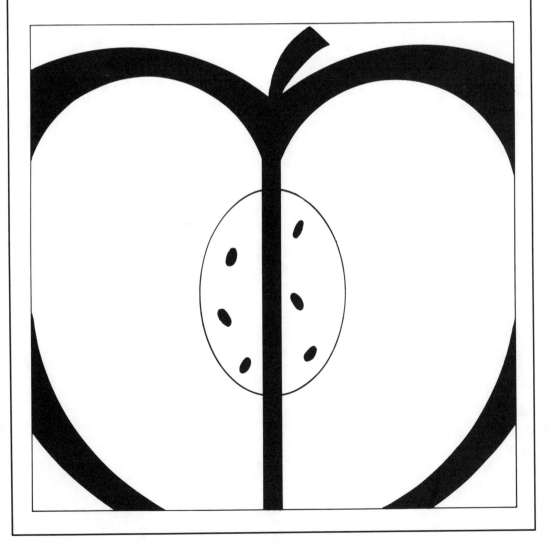

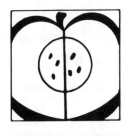

Protein is often considered to be the most important nutrient in our diet. The term was coined from the Greek word *proteios,* meaning "to take first place," but the average American, not wanting to skimp on a good thing, tends to consume far more protein than is really necessary. What often goes unrealized is that along with the extra protein comes extra fat and calories—the "baggage" of high-protein food. Thus, instead of being good to ourselves by getting an abundance of protein, we are probably just overeating.

Self-assessment for protein

To evaluate your diet for protein, consider each of the following questions. Record all statements to which you respond "no" in your notebook; this will be your guide to habits that can be improved. Follow the sample on page 172.

DO YOU USUALLY:

	YES	NO
■ Have meatless meals at least two days per week (without red meat, chicken, or fish)?	_____	_____
■ Aim for a variety of vegetables in a meatless meal?	_____	_____
■ Use legumes (beans, peanuts, and peas) of all kinds in cooking?	_____	_____
■ Have low-fat milk or milk products daily?	_____	_____
■ Have at least four servings of whole-grain breads or cereals each day?	_____	_____
■ Keep meat portions small (not more than an average of 3 to 4 ounces per day or 21 to 28 ounces a week)?	_____	_____
■ Have fish and poultry more often than red meat (beef, veal, lamb, pork)?	_____	_____

Facts to consider

■ A primary health concern of a diet high in animal protein stems from the fact that these foods are often high in extra saturated fat, cholesterol, and calories.

■ The average American tends to eat approximately twice the amount of protein generally recommended.

■ Excessive consumption of protein may tax the kidneys, which rid the body of the extra protein nitrogen it does not need.

■ Protein requirements are high during growth, pregnancy, lactation, and stress (e.g., surgery, fever, infection, injury).

■ Meatless meals tend to provide a better assortment of nutrients because a wider variety of foods is necessary to replace the meat protein.

■ A totally vegetarian diet can provide enough protein when care is taken to balance the essential amino acids provided by certain foods.

■ A totally vegetarian diet (no red meats, chicken, fish, milk, cheese, or eggs) is inadequate in Vitamin B_{12} and needs to be supplemented with this vitamin.

☐ About protein

It is no wonder that protein has been lauded as a first-rate nutrient, for its main function is to maintain body tissues and support growth. There is some protein in every cell of the body, and it comprises 50 percent of the body's dry weight. In addition, protein:

- Contributes to a variety of essential body secretions, lubricants, and fluids. For instance, mucus and milk contain protein, as do some hormones.

- Contains enzymes and hormones that are important in regulating body functions.

- Plays a role in the body's immune system. Antibodies to specific disease are made up of protein.

- Comprises the hard and insoluble coverings of the body such as hair, skin, and nails.

Most of the protein in our bodies is found in the muscle tissue, but it is also distributed in soft tissues, bones, teeth, blood, and other body fluids. In other words, it is just about everywhere.

Protein is made up of large clusters of amino acids and, like fats and carbohydrates, contains carbon, hydrogen, and oxygen. However, protein also contains nitrogen; it is only through protein foods that we obtain this important element. In addition, protein foods contribute sulfur, phosphorus, iron, and cobalt to the diet.

Our bodies can produce many of the twenty-three amino acids that make up proteins; however, eight, or possibly nine, cannot be made in the body and must be supplied from the foods we eat. It is for this reason that they are called "essential" amino acids. Because all the necessary amino acids must be present at the same time in order to make new proteins, a short supply of any one can limit protein synthesis and the food will be utilized as calories instead.

The ability of our bodies to use foods to make protein is based on several factors.

1 The ability of the body to make protein depends on whether or not the diet contains enough calories to fulfill the body's energy requirements. If calorie intake from carbohydrate and fat is low, the body is forced to use protein food for energy instead of building and repairing tissues. This is one of the primary problems of malnutrition in developing nations, where the real problem is a shortage of calories. In many cases, if more calories came from carbohydrates and fats, there would be adequate protein to support normal growth and development.

2   How often protein is eaten is important. Since protein cannot be stored in the body, as can fats and carbohydrates, it is best to eat protein daily. Ideally, the balance of amino acids needed to make protein should be supplied at each meal.

3   Proteins eaten in excess of the body's requirements for protein synthesis will be utilized as a calorie source. A lot of expensive protein calories are being wasted in this way, for the average American adult eats twice the amount of protein generally recommended.

4   Protein production depends on whether or not the foods consumed provide a balance of essential amino acids. As stated earlier, unless the proportions of amino acids are right, they are likely to be wasted as a protein source. A balanced supply should be eaten at every meal, or if eaten at different meals, they should be within four to six hours of each other.

Most of us are aware of the protein-rich animal foods such as meat, milk, and eggs. What many of us overlook, however, is the wealth of proteins found in vegetable sources, such as beans, peas, and grains. Many of the vegetables we commonly look upon as being "starchy," such as rice, are also a source of protein and do not contain the saturated fat and cholesterol so often found in animal products.

While it is true that such *individual* vegetable protein foods (with the exception of soybeans) are not as well-balanced with respect to essential amino acids as are animal proteins, a balance can be attained by eating *several* vegetable foods together. By doing so, the amino acids deficient in one vegetable source are supplied by another. For example, rice and beans together supply a good balance of amino acids, whereas each alone is low in certain amino acids. Combining foods in this manner is called "complementing proteins." Although there has been a great deal of discussion and a lot of confusion about complementing proteins, it needn't worry you. The average adult who gets an adequate amount of calories and who eats a variety of foods will be getting plenty of protein.

Of greater concern in American eating habits is the *overconsumption* of animal protein foods. While total protein in our diets has changed little during the past sixty-five years, there has been a shift in food sources. In the beginning of the century Americans received half of their protein from animal sources and half from vegetable sources. We now obtain more than two-thirds of our protein from animal products. Along with these changes has come an increase in saturated fats and cholesterol in the American diet.

Overeating animal foods is a costly proposition from the viewpoints of both health and economics. Raising animals for food consumption is expensive, and in a world of shrinking natural resources we would do well to limit the amount of these foods in our diet.

☐ **Making changes**

Balance the protein in your diet to provide sufficient, rather than excessive, amounts. The sections that follow will help you to do so by outlining how to:

- Estimate your protein requirements.
- Choose foods to meet your requirements.
- Plan meatless meals.

ESTIMATE YOUR PROTEIN REQUIREMENTS

Many people are surprised when they realize how easily protein requirements are met. The Food and Nutrition Board of the National Research Council has established Recommended Dietary Allowances (RDA) for protein based on age and weight (see pages 144–45). In order to realize your requirements, use the following formula set by the council.

Protein grams/day = body weight in kilograms (kg)* x .8 grams
OR
My weight in pounds ____ ÷ 2.2 = ____ (wt. in kg) × .8 = ____ grams
of protein
per day

For example:
A woman weighing 58 kg (128 pounds) requires 46 grams of protein/day:
58 kg x .8 grams = 46 grams per day

The requirement for a man weighing 70 kg (154 pounds) is 56 grams of protein:
70 kg x .8 grams = 56 grams per day

*To obtain weight in kilograms, divide your weight in pounds by 2.2.

FOODS TO MEET PROTEIN REQUIREMENTS

Note that it does not take a great deal of food to meet these requirements. The list below shows portions of food that are equal to approximately 6 grams of protein.

½ cup	Dried beans or peas (cooked)
2 slices	Whole-wheat bread
¼ cup	Cottage cheese
1 oz	Cheese—cheddar, swiss, mozzarella, etc.
2 cups	Farina or corn grits (cooked)
¾ cup	Skim milk
¼ cup	Nuts (walnuts, almonds, peanuts)
1 cup	Pasta (cooked)
2 tbsp	Peanut butter
1 cup	Oatmeal (cooked)
¼ cup	Seeds (pumpkin, sunflower, sesame)
¼ cup	Wheat germ
½ cup	Plain, low-fat yogurt
1 oz	Lean meat, fish, poultry (cooked)
⅔ piece	Tofu (⅔ of piece that is 2½″ x 2¾″ x 1″)

The woman weighing 58 kilograms can achieve her protein requirement of 46 grams with:

PORTION	PROTEIN (grams)
1 cup plain low-fat yogurt	12
2 slices whole-wheat bread	6
2 tbsp peanut butter	6
3 oz lean meat	18
¾ cup skim milk	6
	48

The 70-kilogram man requiring 56 grams of protein can meet his needs with:

PORTION	PROTEIN (grams)
1 cup cooked farina	**6**
1 cup skim milk	**8**
2 slices whole wheat bread	**6**
¾ cup cottage cheese	**18**
¼ cup wheat germ	**6**
½ cup cooked beans	**6**
1 cup cooked pasta	**6**
	56

Now compare this amount of protein with a more typical pattern in the American diet.

PORTION	PROTEIN (grams)
2 eggs	**12**
4 oz hamburger	**24**
¼ cup peanuts	**6**
10 oz steak	**60**
2 oz cheese	**12**
	114 (or 204% of the average protein requirement)

With just these few high-protein foods, more than twice the amount of protein required would be eaten, in addition to the extra fat and calories that go along with these foods. You can reduce these extra calorie- and fat-carriers in your diet by having protein portions to *meet* requirements and not exceed them.

CUT DOWN ON MEAT

Overeating meat is the most common way to overeat protein. Meat is often eaten twice a day and portion sizes tend to be large as well. Ten-ounce steaks, quarter-pound hamburgers, and half-pound servings of roast beef are common. Cutting down on frequency as well as portion sizes will greatly reduce extra protein, fat, and calories in your diet.

Most of us are completely unaware of portion sizes. It is important to learn how to judge the size of a serving. Calorie tables often refer to 3 ounces of cooked meat. Average portions, however, are usually much larger than this.

To help estimate serving sizes of meats, study the illustrations below and on the following pages. Each illustration represents the *actual size* of a 3-ounce serving of cooked, lean meat (without bone). This portion before cooking would weigh approximately 4 ounces.

Hamburger (lean)
One 3-ounce cooked patty this size:
about **185 calories.**

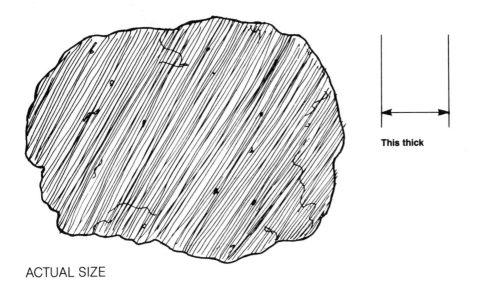

This thick

ACTUAL SIZE

Round steak (lean only)
One 3-ounce cooked piece this size:
about **160 calories.**

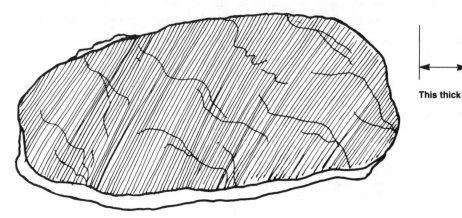

This thick

ACTUAL SIZE

Veal cutlet (trimmed)
One 3-ounce cooked cutlet this size:
about **185 calories.**

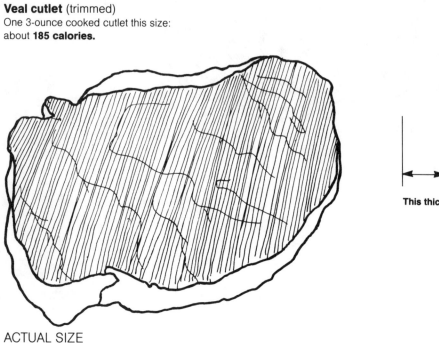

This thick

ACTUAL SIZE

Roast beef round (lean only)
Two slices this size totaling 3 ounces cooked:
about **140 calories.**

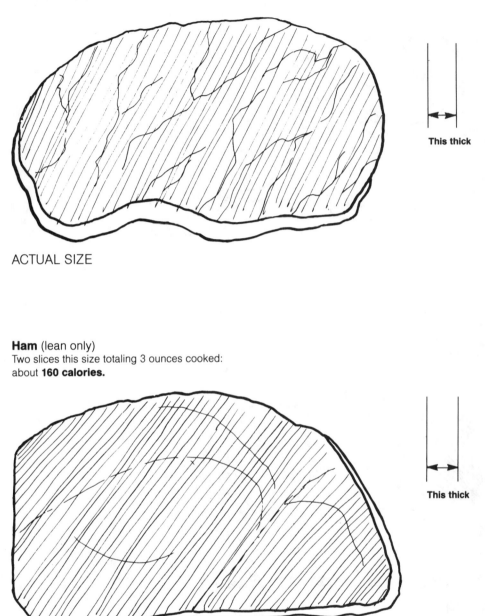

This thick

ACTUAL SIZE

Ham (lean only)
Two slices this size totaling 3 ounces cooked:
about **160 calories.**

This thick

ACTUAL SIZE

Lamb chop (lean only)
Two chops this size (fat removed) totaling 3 ounces cooked:
about **160 calories.**

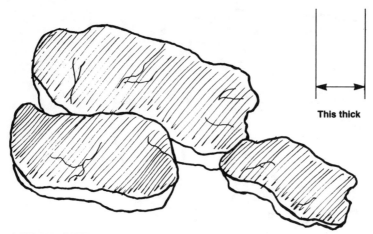

This thick

ACTUAL SIZE

Meat loaf
Two slices this size totaling 3 ounces cooked:
about **170 calories.**

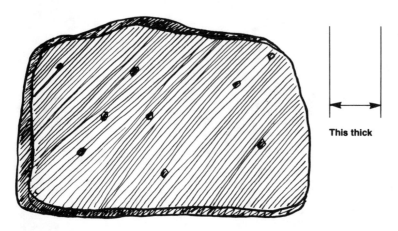

This thick

ACTUAL SIZE

Roast turkey

Two slices of light meat this size totaling 3 ounces cooked:
about **150 calories.**
Two slices of dark meat this size totaling 3 ounces cooked:
about **175 calories.**

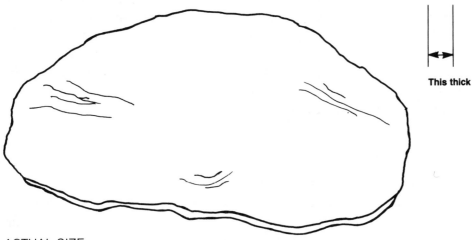

This thick

ACTUAL SIZE

Pork chop (lean only)

Two chops this size (fat removed) totaling 3 ounces cooked:
about **230 calories.**

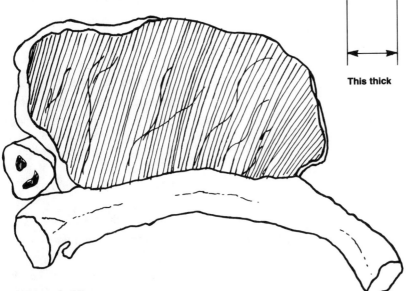

This thick

ACTUAL SIZE

You may be surprised at how small these portions appear. Most of us eat much larger meat portions than these.

If the answers to your self-assessment and a study of these portion sizes reveal that you are eating too much meat, consider some ways of cutting down. There are several options. One is to eat smaller portions of meat but to have it as often as you do now. Another is to keep eating larger portions, but limit the number of times per week you eat meat, filling in with meatless meals. Of course, you can do a little of both. Smaller portions *and* some meatless meals is a sure way of reducing the total amount of meat each week. A reasonable goal is to limit meat to 21 to 28 ounces per week (or about a pound and a half per week).

EAT MEATLESS MEALS SEVERAL TIMES A WEEK

Having meatless meals several times a week is an effective way to reduce extra protein, fat, and calories. The essential thing to learn is that you are replacing the high-quality, complete protein in meat with other protein sources that may be incomplete. In other words, they may be missing or low in one or more of the essential amino acids needed by the body. Knowing how to combine or complement different protein sources is the key to replacing meat protein. For example, rice and beans eaten together supply a good balance of amino acids, whereas each alone is low in certain amino acids. The following table lists combinations that result in complete protein.

PROTEIN COMBINATIONS		FOOD CHOICES
Grain products + peas, beans, or lentils	=	Rice and bean dish
		Garbanzos and corn bread
		Lentil-rice loaf
		Rice and soy grits
		Wheat and soy bread
Milk + grain products	=	Lasagna made with meatless tomato sauce, skim-milk mozzarella, and parmesan cheese
		Yogurt and barley soup
		Ricotta cheese spread and whole-grain bread
Peas, beans, or lentils + sesame seeds	=	Garbanzos, sesame vegetable sauce
		Tofu (or soybean curd) and sesame seeds (as part of a salad)
		Pea soup and sesame muffins

ADDITIONAL SUGGESTIONS

With your meatless meals, try to:

- Have yogurt dressing, cold peas, beans, and toasted seeds in your salads.

- Add nonfat dry milk or soy flour to baked goods and cereals.

- Use nuts, seeds, soy grits, and low-fat cheese on grain dishes.

- Include low-fat dairy products in your meal:

HAVE	INSTEAD OF
Low-fat milk (skim or 1%)	Whole milk, cream, or coffee creamers
Low-fat cottage cheese	High-fat cheeses
Skim-milk cheese (skim-milk ricotta, skim-milk mozzarella)	High-fat cheeses
Low-fat buttermilk	Whole milk or whole-milk buttermilk
Low-fat yogurt	Whole-milk yogurt

- Increase the use of whole-grain cereals and breads in your diet:

HAVE	INSTEAD OF
Whole-grain bread	White bread
Whole-grain cereals (oatmeal, millet, rye)	Presweetened refined cereals
Brown rice	White rice
Soy and whole-wheat flour	White flour

We are not suggesting that everyone become a vegetarian; however, having at least some meatless meals can help minimize several dietary excesses as well as introduce an exciting new dimension to food choices.

Part 6

Sodium:
the hidden nutrient

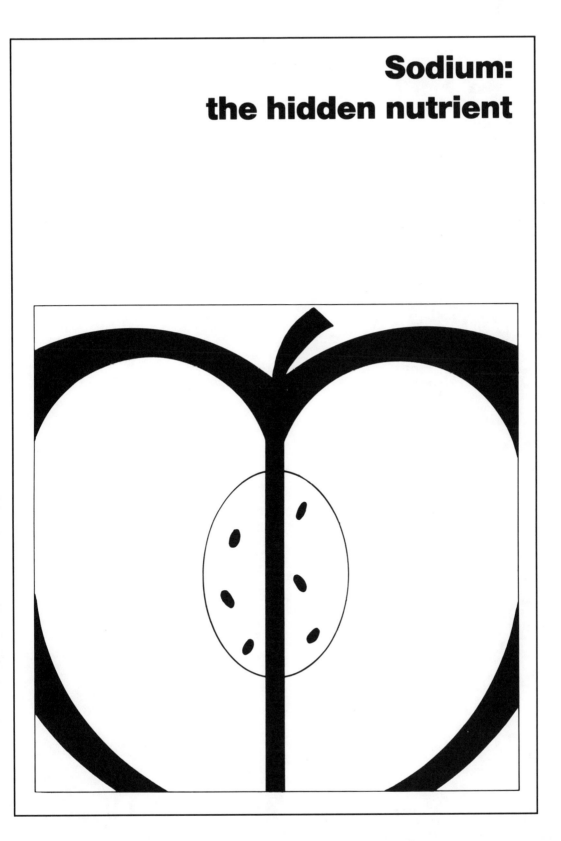

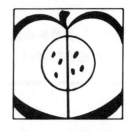

Another problem of excess in our diets has to do with the sodium that we add to our foods. The most familiar source of sodium is table salt, or sodium chloride, which is 40 percent sodium. It creeps into our foods from many sources—at the table, in cooking, and in processed foods.

Sodium is an important mineral in the body, for it helps to regulate water, to balance acids in blood and urine, and to aid absorption of nutrients across cell membranes. It is also involved in muscle contraction and proper activity of the nervous system.

While sodium depletion can occur as a result of excessive vomiting, diarrhea, burns, or excessive sweating, most of us are eating too much rather than too little. It is estimated that Americans consume approximately ten times the amount needed by the body. Although the body is very efficient at regulating body fluids, habitual heavy use of salt may upset this system and result in hypertension and other serious health problems. Retention of fluid may lead to swelling of the ankles, or for those with impaired cardiac function, it can actually cause heart failure.

Self-assessment for sodium

Much of the sodium in our foods is "hidden." Assess your diet for this mineral by answering the following questions. Record all statements to which you answered "no" in your notebook, following the sample on page 172.

DO YOU USUALLY:

	YES	NO
■ Taste your food before salting it?	___	___
■ Use salt sparingly or not at all at the table?	___	___
■ Limit salty foods by reading food labels for added salt or sodium?	___	___
■ Choose snacks of nuts or pretzels that are unsalted?	___	___
■ Have salty luncheon meats (liverwurst, franks, salami, bologna, etc.) not more than once a week?	___	___
■ Go sparingly with salty sauces such as ketchup, soy sauce, or barbecue sauce?	___	___
■ Eat fresh or unsalted frozen vegetables rather than canned vegetables?	___	___
■ Order Chinese food without MSG?	___	___
■ Have canned or frozen entrees not more than twice a week?	___	___
■ Go sparingly with salty snacks such as bouillon, pickles, or olives?	___	___
■ Have only an occasional serving (not more than twice a week) of commercially prepared bouillon, broths, and other soups?	___	___

Facts to consider

■ Diets high in sodium tend to increase blood pressure in individuals prone to hypertension and increase fluid retention in others.

■ Sodium can be found in many processed foods. Learn to read labels for sodium or salt content.

■ Buying fresh or plain, frozen vegetables rather than processed foods can often save a great deal of sodium. For example, canned vegetables may have forty times the sodium of fresh vegetables.

■ A sudden excess of sodium intake can cause headaches and mental confusion. This occurs most often from oriental food containing MSG and has been referred to as the "Chinese restaurant syndrome."

Be aware of salty foods

Processed meats:
bologna, salami, franks,
bacon, corned beef

Canned vegetables

Potato chips, pretzels,
salted nuts

Relish, horseradish

Soy sauce, ketchup

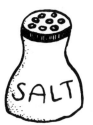

Cheeses

Commercial soups

Pickles, sauerkraut,
olives

Sardines, anchovies,
marinated herring

Frozen entrees

☐ About sodium

Sodium in our diet comes not only from the salt we add to foods ourselves, but also from the salt and other sodium compounds (such as baking soda and monosodium glutamate) added to commercially prepared foods. In fact, salt is one of the leading food additives (after sugar)! The following list identifies some of the most important sodium compounds added to foods.*

- *Salt (sodium chloride).* This is used in cooking or at the table, as well as in canning and processing.

- *Monosodium glutamate (also called MSG).* MSG is sold under several brand names and is a seasoning used in home, restaurant, and hotel cooking, and in many packaged, canned, or frozen foods. It is often used generously in oriental foods.

- *Baking powder.* Baking powder is used to leaven quick breads and cakes.

- *Baking soda (sodium bicarbonate).* Baking soda is used to leaven breads and cakes; it is sometimes added to vegetables in cooking or used as an "alkalizer" for indigestion.

- *Brine (table salt and water).* Brine is used in processed foods to inhibit growth of bacteria, as in corned beef, pastrami, pickles, and sauerkraut; in cleaning or blanching vegetables and fruits; and in freezing and canning certain foods.

- *Disodium phosphate.* This is present in some quick-cooking cereals and processed cheeses. It is used as an emulsifier in some cheeses and as a buffer to adjust acidity in chocolate products, beverages, sauces, and quick-cooking cereals.

- *Sodium alginate.* Sodium alginate is used in many chocolate milks and ice creams for smooth texture.

- *Sodium benzoate.* Sodium benzoate is used as a preservative in many condiments, such as relishes, sauces, and salad dressings.

- *Sodium hydroxide.* Sodium hydroxide is used in food processing to soften and loosen skins of ripe olives, hominy, and certain fruits and vegetables.

- *Sodium propionate.* Sodium propionate is used in pasteurized cheeses and in some breads and cakes to inhibit growth of mold.

- *Sodium sulfite.* Sodium sulfite is used to bleach certain fruits in which an artificial color is desired, such as maraschino cherries and glazed or crystallized fruit; it is also used as a preservative in some dried fruits, such as prunes.

*Reprinted by permission of the American Heart Association: "Your Mild Sodium-Restricted Diet," 1975, pp. 8–9.

While sodium is found in all of these products, it is the first five that are the major contributors of sodium to our diet.

☐ Making changes

The primary goal is to limit consumption of sodium. Like so many other elements of our diet, we eat too much of it. To begin to cut down, consider the following guidelines:

- To condition your taste to less sodium, gradually reduce the amount of salt you use at the table. Have your goal be to avoid adding any salt at the table. The conditioning takes approximately two weeks.

- To limit the amount of salt added when preparing foods, start cutting down by using just half the amount of salt called for in recipes.

- Be aware of "hidden" sodium in commercially prepared foods. Especially learn to avoid foods with MSG added to them.

- Season foods with herbs and spices instead of salt. (See the next page.)

- Avoid or limit high-sodium foods. Use the list below as a guide.

HAVE	INSTEAD OF
Fresh or frozen vegetables (read labels for added salt; frozen vegetables vary in the amount of added salt)	Canned vegetables, sauerkraut, pickles, and foods prepared in brine
Whole-grain or enriched breads	Breads, rolls, and crackers with salted tops
Fresh potatoes	Potato chips, canned potatoes
Unsalted nuts and pretzels	Salted nuts and pretzels
All fresh meats, poultry, fish, and shellfish	Cured, salted, canned, or smoked meats, poultry, and fish (e.g., corned beef, ham, bacon, luncheon meats, frankfurters, other sausages, sardines, anchovies, and marinated herring)
Unsalted or lightly salted homemade soup	Bouillon, canned or commercially prepared soups (especially Chinese soups)
Seasonings or spices and herbs	Soy sauce, ketchup, garlic salt, onion salt, MSG, prepared mustard

Season with herbs and spices instead of salt

MEAT, FISH, POULTRY, AND EGGS

Beef—Allspice, basil, bay leaf, cardamom, chives, curry, garlic, mace, marjoram, dry mustard, nutmeg, onion, oregano, paprika, parsley, pepper, green peppers, sage, savory, tarragon, thyme, turmeric

Pork—Basil, cardamom, cloves, curry, dill, garlic, mace, marjoram, dry mustard, oregano, onion, parsley, pepper, rosemary, sage, thyme, turmeric

Lamb—Basil, curry, dill, garlic, mace, marjoram, mint, onion, oregano, parsley, pepper, rosemary, thyme, turmeric

Veal—Basil, bay leaf, curry, dill, garlic, ginger, mace, marjoram, oregano, paprika, parsley, peaches, pepper, rosemary, sage, savory, tarragon, thyme, turmeric

Chicken or turkey—Allspice, basil, bay leaf, cardamom, cumin, curry, garlic, mace, marjoram, mushrooms, dry mustard, paprika, parsley, pepper, pineapple sauce, rosemary, sage, savory, tarragon, thyme, turmeric

Fish—Bay leaf, chives, coriander, curry, dill, garlic, lemon juice, mace, marjoram, mushrooms, dry mustard, onion, oregano, paprika, parsley, pepper, green peppers, sage, savory, tarragon, thyme, turmeric

Eggs—Basil, chili powder, chives, cumin, curry, mace, marjoram, dry mustard, onion, paprika, parsley, pepper, green peppers, rosemary, savory, tarragon, thyme

VEGETABLES

Asparagus—Caraway seed, dry mustard, nutmeg, sesame seed

Broccoli—Oregano, tarragon

Cabbage—Basil, caraway seed, cinnamon, dill, mace, dry mustard, nutmeg, savory, tarragon

Carrots—Chili powder, cinnamon, ginger, mace, marjoram, mint, nutmeg, parsley, poppy seed, thyme

Cauliflower—Caraway seed, curry, dill, mace, nutmeg, rosemary, savory, tarragon

Corn—Chili powder, chives, curry, parsley

Green beans—Basil, bay leaf, dill, cinnamon, lemon juice, mace, marjoram, nutmeg, onion, oregano, rosemary, sesame seed

Peas—Cinnamon, dill, mace, marjoram, mint, mushrooms, dry mustard, onion, oregano, parsley, green peppers, poppy seed, savory, thyme

Potatoes—Caraway seed, chives, dill, mace, mint, oregano, onion, parsley, poppy seed, thyme

Squash—Basil, ginger, mace, marjoram, oregano

Sweet potato—Allspice, cardamom, ginger

Tomatoes—Basil, chives, dill, marjoram, oregano, parsley, sage, tarragon, thyme

MIXED SEASONINGS—
Seasoning mixtures without salt are available. Examples are Bell's Poultry Seasoning, Fines Herbes, Italian Herbs, Bouquet Garni. A guideline for use is ¼ to ½ teaspoon of seasoning per 4 servings.

From: "Add Flavor to Your Sodium-Restricted Diet," New York State Department of Health.

Sodium is necessary in our diet, but the requirement is for an amount much smaller than we are accustomed to. The easiest way to cut down on sodium is to cut down on salt. Experimenting with alternative herbs and spices can be a pleasant way to improve the diet.

Part 7

Vitamins and minerals: the vulnerable nutrients

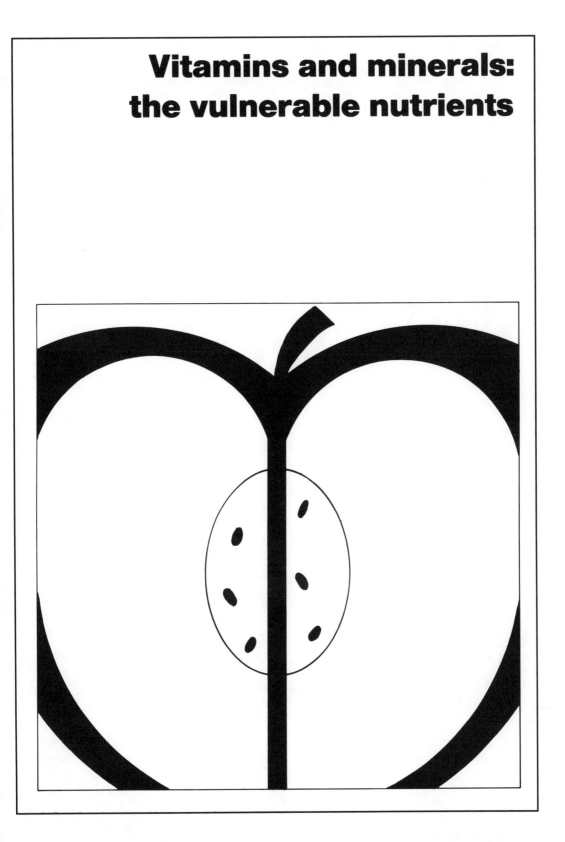

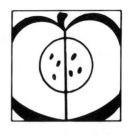

Despite the overconsumption of food in the United States, the diets of some Americans may still be low in certain nutrients. Our bountiful food supply easily provides enough calories, fat, carbohydrates, and protein, but unless foods are chosen, stored, and prepared carefully, essential vitamins and minerals may be missing from our diet.

Although vitamins and minerals are needed in relatively small quantities compared with fat, protein, and carbohydrates, they are easily lost from foods for several reasons:

- Overprocessing often results in the loss of important nutrients. Even fortification and enrichment do not make up for all the losses of nutrients that occur during the commercial processing of foods.

- Prolonged storage depletes foods of vitamins. Vitamin C is particularly vulnerable to this type of destruction.

- Careless food preparation can cause substantial losses. Vitamins and minerals may be peeled, soaked, and cooked away, unless care is taken to minimize such losses.

A great deal happens to food from the time it leaves the farm until it reaches our tables. It is worth the effort to take care in selection, storage, and preparation in order to get the most from foods.

We are often told that eating a varied, balanced diet is the key to supplying our bodies with the necessary nutrients. While this is true for the average, healthy person, it is not as simple as it sounds. Variety of foods means not only foods from different food groups but also variety in the supply, form, and preparation of foods. Because different foods contain different nutrients and because vitamin and mineral losses vary according to the method of food storage and preparation, it is important to eat as many kinds of foods as possible.

Consider your habits in selecting and preparing foods. Are you doing the most you can to get the vitamins and minerals your body needs?

Self-assessment for vitamins and minerals

Careful food selection, food storage, and preparation are the keys to providing essential vitamins and minerals to the body. Assess your habits by answering the following questions. Record all statements to which you answered "no" in your notebook as an indication of those habits you need to acquire. Follow the sample on page 172.

☐ Food selection

DO YOU USUALLY:

	YES	NO
■ Have at least four servings of whole-grain bread and cereals a day?	____	____
■ Use whole-grain flour rather than white, refined flour?	____	____
■ Have brown rice rather than white rice?	____	____
■ Have *at least* one serving a day of fruits and vegetables rich in vitamin C (e.g., oranges, grapefruits, strawberries, cantaloupe, tomato juice, potato, broccoli, spinach, green pepper)?	____	____
■ Have two or more servings per day of dark green, leafy, and yellow vegetables (e.g., broccoli, carrots, escarole, spinach, sweet potatoes, winter squash)?	____	____
■ Vary choice of vegetables between fresh and frozen products?	____	____
■ Carefully select produce for quality and freshness?	____	____
■ Make certain to have iron-rich foods daily (e.g., lean meats, legumes, whole grains, and green, leafy vegetables)?	____	____
■ Have two servings of low-fat milk or milk products a day (1 serving = 1 cup of skim milk or 1 cup plain yogurt)?	____	____

■ Have only occasionally or not at all highly refined, empty-calorie foods (such as sodas, candy, sugar, alcohol)?   _____ _____

■ Eat a variety of different fruits and vegetables?   _____ _____

☐ Food storage and preparation

DO YOU USUALLY:

■ Use a minimal amount of water in cooking?   _____ _____

■ Steam, stir fry, or pressure cook vegetables rather than boil them?   _____ _____

■ When cooking vegetables in water, add them to boiling water?   _____ _____

■ Use the liquid in which food is prepared instead of discarding it?   _____ _____

■ Consider vegetables "done" while they are still firm rather than mushy?   _____ _____

■ Minimize mashing, shredding, or chopping fruits and vegetables?   _____ _____

■ Cook or serve immediately foods that have been mashed, shredded, or chopped?   _____ _____

■ Avoid allowing foods to stand exposed to heat, light, and air?   _____ _____

■ Avoid prolonged storage of fresh produce?   _____ _____

■ Store vegetable oil in a cool, dark place?   _____ _____

■ Minimize the cooking time of meats to preserve nutrients?   _____ _____

■ Avoid using baking soda when cooking green vegetables?   _____ _____

Facts to consider

- Cooking and soaking foods in water leaches out vitamin C, the B-complex vitamins, and minerals.

- Minimizing heat and cooking time helps preserve vitamin C and certain B vitamins (thiamin, pyridoxine, vitamin B_{12}, folic acid, and riboflavin).

- Exposure to light destroys folic acid, riboflavin, pyridoxine, vitamin B_{12}, vitamin C, vitamin E, vitamin A, and vitamin K.

- Oxidation from exposure to oxygen in the air can cause the destruction of vitamin A, carotene, vitamin C, vitamin E, vitamin K, thiamin, pyridoxine, biotin, and folic acid.

- Baking soda tends to destroy folic acid, thiamin, and ascorbic acid by creating an alkaline medium.

- According to government studies, many people do not get adequate amounts of vitamins A and C and the mineral calcium.

- Women during their reproductive years require more iron than men, and need to eat more foods rich in iron.

- Eating foods rich in vitamin C along with foods rich in iron will improve the absorption of iron.

- Whole grains are rich in trace minerals that are missing in refined flours—even when these flours are enriched.

- Too many highly refined foods are likely to result in a diet that is deficient in vitamins and minerals.

☐ About vitamins

Vitamins are organic compounds that are essential in many of the chemical reactions in the body. Vitamins do not supply energy or serve as part of the body structure (as do minerals and proteins). Rather they act with enzyme systems in initiating and giving impetus to many body functions such as freeing energy from carbohydrate, fat, and protein, detoxifying poisonous substances, enabling blood to clot, and maintaining healthy teeth and bones.

Vitamins must be supplied to the body because we do not manufacture them. They are grouped as either fat-soluble (those that dissolve in fats and oils) or water-soluble (those that dissolve in water). The fat-soluble vitamins (A, D, E, and K) can be stored in the body in almost unlimited amounts, even to the point of toxic levels. This is especially true of vitamins A and D. On the other hand, a continuously low intake may not show up for many months.

The water-soluble vitamins include the B-complex vitamins, vitamin C, and folic acid. They are found in fruits, vegetables, whole grains, and meats. They cannot be stored in the body to any great extent and are particularly vulnerable to destruction during storage and preparation; therefore, they need to be supplied regularly to the body.

☐ About minerals

The body requires many different types of minerals to function normally, and they all must be supplied from our food and drink. Some of the minerals, such as calcium, are required in larger amounts to make up the hard body structures such as bones and teeth. On the other hand, minerals such as zinc, iron, chromium, copper, and others are needed in only trace amounts in order to maintain normal body functions. Besides making up the bony structures of the body, minerals are also involved in the normal functioning of nerves and muscles, in the activation of enzymes, and, in the case of iron, in the transport of oxygen.

About vitamins

Vitamin	Major body functions	Results of deficiency
Vitamin A Retinol	For healthy skin and linings of the mouth, nose, throat, digestive and urinary tracts, and for vision in dim light	Night and glare blindness; permanent blindness; rough, dry skin; retards growth; mental retardation
Vitamin B_1 Thiamin	Coenzyme in reactions involving removal of carbon dioxide; essential for growth, normal appetite, digestion, and healthy nerves	Poor appetite, constipation, irritability, insomnia, abnormal fatigue, beriberi
Vitamin B_2 Riboflavin	For cellular enzyme systems that help release energy from food	Photophobia (eyes unusually sensitive to light); cracks in the corners of mouth; red, scaly areas around the nose

Vitamin B_6
  Pyridoxine,
  Pyridoxal,
  Pyridoxamine
	For the metabolism and synthesis of amino acids, fat and carbohydrate metabolism, central nervous system activity, hemoglobin synthesis	No specific, definable symptoms except those similar to the other B vitamins

Vitamin B_{12}	For metabolic processes in all cells, specifically for red blood cell formation	Pernicious anemia, megaloblastic anemia
Folic Acid	For amino acid metabolism and blood cell formation; helps in synthesis of nucleic acids vital to all nuclei	Macrocytic anemia, diarrhea, glossitis (smooth tongue)
Niacin	For normal functioning of tissues of the skin, gastrointestinal tract, and the nervous system; functions with other vitamins in converting carbohydrate into energy	Pellagra: swollen, beefy red tongue, loss of appetite, diarrhea, symmetrical dermatitis, lassitude, anxiety, depression
Pantothenic Acid	Essential component of enzyme systems in the metabolism of carbohydrate, fat, and protein	No conclusive clinical symptoms
Biotin	For helping in the intermediary metabolism of fat, carbohydrate, and protein and in fatty acid synthesis	Experimentally induced only: mild eczema-like dermatitis, nausea, loss of appetite, anemia, depression, sleeplessness, muscle pain

Results of excess	Good food sources	Losses in food preparation
Headache, vomiting, peeling of skin, anorexia, swelling, long bones, loss of body hair, enlargement of liver and spleen	Liver, dark green leafy and yellow vegetables (broccoli, carrots, winter squash), apricots, cantaloupe, milk, cheese, butter, fortified margarine, eggs	Slowly destroyed by air and light; cooking losses minimal
None reported	Pork, lean meat, poultry, liver, heart, kidney, whole-grain and enriched cereals and breads, wheat germ, fish, yeast, legumes	Readily destroyed in heat, air; water-soluble, heat-stable in acid
None reported	Milk, liver, kidney, heart, lean meats, eggs, dark leafy greens, enriched bread and cereal	Stable in heat for cooking; water-soluble, unstable in light or alkali
None reported	Whole-grain cereals, wheat germ, meat, fish, vegetables	Considered stable in oxygen, heat, and light; water-soluble
None reported	Liver, kidney, meat, eggs, milk, dairy foods	Unstable in air, light, acid, and alkali; water-soluble
None reported	Green leafy vegetables, liver, kidney, lean beef, wheat, eggs, fish, dry beans, lentils, cowpeas, asparagus, broccoli, collards	Unstable in heat and air
Flushing, burning, and tingling around neck, face, and hands	Lean meats, liver, fish, whole-grain and enriched cereals and breads, eggs, legumes	Stable in heat, light, air, acid, and alkali; water-soluble
None reported	In all plant and animal foods; best sources are eggs, kidney, liver, salmon, and yeast	Unstable in acid, alkali, and heat; water-soluble
None reported	Liver, kidney, eggs, mushrooms, peanuts, milk, most vegetables, bananas, grapefruit, tomatoes, watermelon, strawberries	Stable in heat, light, and air; water-soluble

About vitamins (continued)

Vitamin	Major body functions	Results of deficiency
Vitamin C Ascorbic Acid	For formation of intercellular substances, for healthy connective tissue, cartilage, bones, teeth, blood vessels	Spongy, bleeding gums; tendency to bruise easily; painful, swollen joints; scurvy
Vitamin D Cholecalciferol	For calcium and phosphorus absorption and utilization in formation of bones and teeth	Soft bones, bowed legs, poor teeth, rickets
Vitamin E Tocopherol	For the maintenance of structure and integrity of cellular and subcellular membranes; protects tissue fats and vitamin A from destructive oxidation	Extremely rare, mostly in premature infants: edema, irritability, anemia
Vitamin K	For synthesis of precoagulation factors (prothrombin)	Slow blood clotting, hemorrhagic disease of the newborn

From: Marcella Katz, ''Vitamins, Food and Your Health,'' Public Affairs Pamphlet no. 465, and Neven S. Scrimshaw and Vernon R. Young, ''The Requirements of Human Nutrition,'' *Scientific American* (September 1976), pp. 50–64.

Marie V. Krause and L. Kathleen Mahon, *Food, Nutrition and Diet Therapy,* 6th ed. (Philadelphia: W.B. Saunders Co., 1979).

Results of excess	Good food sources	Losses in food preparation
Relatively nontoxic; possibility of kidney stones	Oranges, grapefruit, strawberries, cantaloupe, tomatoes, peppers, potatoes, cabbage, broccoli, greens	Destroyed by heat, light, air, drying, and aging; water-soluble
Vomiting, diarrhea, loss of weight, kidney damage	Vitamin D fortified milk, fish, liver oils, some in milk fat, egg yolk, salmon, tuna, sardines	Stable in heat, oxygen, aging, and storage under normal conditions
Relatively nontoxic	Vegetable oils, whole-grain cereals, wheat germ, leafy vegetables, nuts, beans	Stable in heat, acid, fat, alkali, and oxygen
Relatively nontoxic; synthetic forms at high doses may cause jaundice	Leafy vegetables, soybean oil, other vegetable oils, wheat bran, tomatoes, cauliflower	Stable in heat and oxygen; sensitive to acids and light

About minerals

Mineral	Major body functions	Results of deficiency
Calcium	Bone and tooth formation; blood clotting; nerve transmission	Stunted growth; rickets, osteoporosis; convulsions
Phosphorus	Bone and tooth formation; acid-base balance	Weakness, demineralization of bone; loss of calcium
Sulfur	Constituent of active tissue compounds, cartilage, and tendon	Related to intake and deficiency of sulfur amino acids
Potassium	Acid-base balance; body water balance; nerve function	Muscular weakness; paralysis
Chlorine	Formation of gastric juice; acid-base balance	Muscle cramps; mental apathy; reduced appetite
Sodium	Acid-base balance; body water balance; nerve function	Muscle cramps; mental apathy; reduced appetite
Magnesium	Activates enzymes; involved in protein synthesis	Growth failure; behavioral disturbances; weakness, spasms
Iron	Constituent of hemoglobin and enzymes involved in energy metabolism	Iron-deficiency anemia (weakness, reduced resistance to infection)
Fluorine	May be important in maintenance of bone structure	Higher frequency of tooth decay
Zinc	Constituent of enzymes involved in digestion	Growth failure, lack of sexual maturation, loss of appetite, abnormal glucose tolerance
Copper	Constituent of enzymes associated with iron metabolism	Anemia, bone changes (rare in man)
Silicon Vanadium Tin Nickel	Function unknown (essential for animals)	Not reported in man
Selenium	Functions in close association with vitamin E	Anemia (rare)

Results of excess	Good food sources
Not reported in man	Milk, cheese, dark green vegetables, dried legumes, sardines, shellfish
Erosion of jaw	Milk, cheese, meat, fish, poultry, whole grains, legumes, nuts
Excess sulfur amino acid intake leads to poor growth	Protein foods (meat, fish, poultry, eggs, milk, cheese, legumes, nuts)
Muscular weakness; death	Meats, milk, many fruits, legumes, vegetables
Vomiting	Common table salt, seafood, milk, meat, eggs
High blood pressure	Common table salt, seafood, animal foods, milk, eggs, grains, most foods except fruit
Diarrhea	Whole grains, green leafy vegetables, nuts, meats, milk, legumes
Siderosis; cirrhosis of liver	Liver, lean meats, legumes, whole grains, dark green vegetables, eggs, dark molasses, shrimp, oysters
Mottling of teeth; increased bone density; neurological disturbances	Drinking water, tea, coffee, seafood, rice, soybeans, spinach, gelatin, onions, lettuce
Fever, nausea, vomiting, diarrhea	Milk, liver, shellfish, herring, wheat bran
Wilson's disease (rare metabolic condition)	Drinking water, liver, shellfish, whole grains, cherries, legumes, kidney, poultry, oysters, nuts, chocolate
Industrial exposures: silicon—silicosis; vanadium—lung irritation; tin—vomiting; nickel—acute pneumonitis	Widely distributed in foods
Gastrointestinal disorders; lung irritation	Fish, poultry, meats, grains, milk, vegetables (depending on soil)

About minerals (continued)

Mineral	Major body functions	Results of deficiency
Manganese	Constituent of enzymes involved in fat synthesis	In animals: poor growth, disturbances of nervous system, reproductive abnormalities
Iodine	Constituent of thyroid hormones	Goiter (enlarged thyroid)
Molybdenum	Constituent of some enzymes	Not reported in man
Chromium	Involved in glucose and energy metabolism	Impaired ability to metabolize glucose
Cobalt	Constituent of vitamin B_{12}	Not reported in man

Adapted from: Neven S. Scrimshaw and Vernon R. Young, "The Requirements of Human Nutrition," *Scientific American* (September 1976), p. 64.

Other Reference: Marie V. Krause and L. Kathleen Mahon, *Food, Nutrition and Diet Therapy,* 6th ed. (Philadelphia: W.B. Saunders Co., 1979).

Results of excess	Good food sources
Poisoning in manganese mines: generalized disease of nervous system	Beet greens, blueberries, whole grains, nuts, legumes, fruit, tea
Very high intakes depress thyroid activity	Marine fish and shellfish, dairy products, many vegetables, iodized salt
Inhibition of enzymes	Legumes, cereals, organ meats, dark green leafy vegetables
Occupational exposures: skin and kidney damage	Fats, vegetable oils, meats, clams, whole-grain cereals
Industrial exposure: dermatitis and diseases of red blood cells	Organ and muscle meats, milk, oysters, clams, poultry, milk, variable in grains and vegetables depending on soil

☐ What about megadoses?

Today some people have turned to megadoses of vitamins and minerals as curative and preventive measures for a variety of physical and psychological problems ranging from the common cold to schizophrenia, hyperactivity, and sexual impotence. The attitude seems to be that if a little is good, more might be better, or if it can't hurt, it might help. This is risky thinking, for high doses are potentially harmful. Such problems as altered metabolism, toxic storage, and inaccurate medical laboratory tests have already been identified as some of the consequences.

While megadoses may hold some promise for the future in the treatment of certain diseases, the taking of vitamins and minerals in amounts far exceeding the Recommended Dietary Allowances (see pages 144–45) is not suggested for the general public.

This is not to say that we need not be concerned about supplying our bodies with the necessary nutrients. Quite the contrary—*we should be very concerned.* Many of our foods have been depleted of important vitamins and minerals; it is possible to get more than enough calories yet be deficient in other nutrients. However, we can get the daily requirements of vitamins and minerals in a natural way from a well-balanced diet of properly prepared foods.

The vitamins and minerals have specific yet often interrelated functions in the body. For a more detailed account of these nutrients, see the charts on pages 124–131.

☐ Making changes

Having a diet rich in vitamins and minerals involves some care in the selection, storage, and preparation of your foods. Use the following guidelines to help you get the most out of your meals.

FOOD SELECTION

It is important to start out with vitamin- and mineral-rich foods. Keep the following points in mind when making food choices.

VARIATION

Once again, it must be stressed that variation in food choice is a key to assuring a balance of vitamins and minerals so that one food will supply what another may lack. Even within the same category of food there are wide variations depending upon the season, soil, or growing conditions.

WHOLE FOODS

Have a predominance of foods in your diet that are as close as possible to the original food. In other words, minimize the amount of processed or refined food you choose. Nature has established a wonderful balance of vitamins and minerals in the original food that is never quite as good once the food is processed.

FRESH FOODS
Foods that are fresh and of high quality are usually higher in vitamin content. This is particularly true of fresh fruits and vegetables, which are a rich source of these nutrients.

In selecting vegetables, remember to choose those that are:

- Bright and natural in color.

- Free of decay or discoloration.

- Crisp—not wilted or shriveled.

Remember, too, that the leaves of plants are the richest in nutrients, with flowers intermediate and the stems lowest.

In selecting fresh fruits, choose those that are:

- Free from bruises and blemishes.

- Firm.

- Plump.

- Ideal color.

Check the charts on pages 135–41. They will give you details for fruit and vegetable selection and storage.

FOOD STORAGE

The method used to store foods together with the amount of time they are stored affects the retention of important vitamins.

The longer fruits and vegetables are stored, the more vitamins are destroyed through oxidation. Storage times vary—some vegetables and fruits can stay "fresh" longer than others. For example, carrots can be kept for several months, celery for several weeks, but leafy greens can be kept for only a few days.

Refrigeration or freezing helps to slow the enzyme activity that causes oxidation. Even though a bowl of fruit is lovely to look at, it is best to keep fruits and vegetables in the refrigerator if you plan on storing them for several days. Vegetable oils should also be kept in a cool, dark place to prevent rancidity and to preserve vitamin E.

Riboflavin can be destroyed by light. Store milk, which is high in riboflavin, in cartons or brown bottles to prevent destruction of this nutrient.

FOOD PREPARATION

Food preparation also greatly affects the preservation of vitamins and minerals. Two basic types of losses can occur during food preparation:

- Solution loss, when nutrients are dissolved.

- Destruction, when too much heat or light is present and the vitamins are broken down.

Vitamins can be lost either by solution or destruction, but minerals can only be dissolved—they cannot be destroyed.

Read through the table on pages 142–43 for a detailed description of how vitamins and minerals can be lost.

Guide to selection and storage of fresh vegetables

Vegetable	Selection criteria	Storage
Asparagus	Good green color extending down much of stalk; closed and compact tips; crisp and tender stalk	Do not wash before storing; store in refrigerator in crisper, plastic bags, or plastic containers; use within 2–3 days
Beans (green and wax)	Bright color for the variety; pods that are firm and crisp rather than flabby	Store in the refrigerator in crisper, plastic bags, or plastic containers; use within 1 week
Beets	Fresh-looking tops if still attached; surface that is smooth and deep red; firm and round with slim top root	Remove tops; store in refrigerator in plastic bags or plastic containers; use within 2 weeks
Broccoli	Dark green to purplish color with no trace of yellow in bud clusters; smooth stalks of moderate size with no traces of spoilage	Store in refrigerator in crisper, plastic bags, or plastic containers; use within 3–5 days
Brussels sprouts	Fresh green color void of yellow leaves; tight outer leaves free of injury; tight heads	Store in refrigerator in crisper, plastic bags, or plastic containers; use within 3–5 days
Cabbage	Firm head; fresh color in outer leaves; crisp leaves	Store in the refrigerator in crisper, plastic bags, or plastic containers; use within 1–2 weeks
Carrots	Crisp rather than flabby; good orange color free from sunburned green at top	Remove tops; store in refrigerator in plastic bags or plastic containers; use within 2 weeks
Cauliflower	Uniform creamy white color with no trace of dark discoloration; solid and compact head; fresh leaves if attached	Store in refrigerator in crisper, plastic bags, or plastic containers; use within 1 week
Celery	Crisp stalks with a solid feel; glossy surface on stalk; crisp leaves; no discoloration on inside surface of large outer stalks	Store in refrigerator in crisper, plastic bags, or plastic containers; use within 1 week
Corn	Ear well covered with plump young kernels; fresh husks that are green and unwilted; silks free of decay	Store, unhusked and uncovered, in the refrigerator; use as soon as possible for sweetest flavor
Cucumbers	Firm; moderate size; green color all over	Wash and dry; store in refrigerator in crisper or plastic bags; use within 1 week

Guide to selection and storage of fresh vegetables (continued)

Vegetable	Selection criteria	Storage
Eggplant	Smooth and firm; deep purple skin free of blemishes	Store at cool room temperature, around 60°F (temperatures below 50°F may cause chilling injury); will keep several months at 60°F but only about a week at room temperature
Greens (spinach, kale, collards, chard, beets, turnip, and mustard)	Crisp appearance with good green color typical of the type of green; free from rust and other blemishes; no wilted or decaying areas	Store in refrigerator in crisper or plastic bags; use within 3–5 days
Lettuce	Crisp quality to leaves, with better lettuces being somewhat less crisp but still succulent; free of decay; good color for the variety	Store in crisper in refrigerator, in plastic bags or plastic containers to reduce loss of moisture
Onions, mature	Firm and dry with small necks; no decay	Store at room temperature or slightly cooler, in loosely woven or open mesh container (stored this way, they keep several months; they sprout and decay at high temperatures and in high humidity)
Onions, green	Crisp, bright green tops, free from decay	Store in plastic bags in refrigerator; use within 3–5 days
Parsnips	Smooth and firm; small to medium size; free from blemishes	Remove tops; store in refrigerator in plastic bags or plastic containers; use within 2 weeks
Peas	Crisp pods with fresh green color; pods full but not bulging	Leave in pods and store in refrigerator; use within 3–5 days
Peppers	Firm; deep color; no trace of flabbiness or decay	Wash and dry; store in crisper or in plastic bags in the refrigerator; use within 1 week
Potatoes	Firm; free from sunburned green areas; no decay; skin intact and free from blemishes	To keep for several months, store in a dark, dry place with good ventilation away from any source of heat, with a temperature of about 45°–50°F (light causes greening, which lowers eating quality; high temperatures hasten sprouting and shriveling); if stored at room temperature, use within 1 week

Vegetable	Selection criteria	Storage
Radishes	Medium size; firm and plump; fresh red color	Remove tops; store in refrigerator in plastic bags or plastic containers; use within 2 weeks
Squash (summer)	Well developed with no soft areas; firm; glossy and tender skin	Store in refrigerator in crisper, plastic bags, or plastic containers; use within 3–5 days
Squash (winter)	Well developed with no soft areas; firm; tough and hard skin	Store at cool room temperature, around 60°F (temperatures below 50°F may cause chilling injury); these will keep several months at 60°F but only about 1 week at room temperature
Sweet potatoes	Firm; good color; no signs of decay at ends	Store at cool room temperature, around 60°F (temperatures below 50°F may cause chilling injury); these will keep several months at 60°F but only about 1 week at room temperature
Tomatoes	Smooth; good color for stage of ripeness; firm if not fully ripe, but slightly soft if ripe; free from blemishes	Store ripe tomatoes uncovered in the refrigerator (can be stored this way up to 1 week, depending upon ripeness); keep unripe tomatoes at room temperature away from direct sunlight until they ripen
Turnips	Firm and smooth; free of blemishes	Remove tops; store in refrigerator in plastic bags or plastic containers; use within 2 weeks

Chart adapted from: Margaret McWilliams, *Food Fundamentals,* 2nd ed. (New York: Wiley, 1974), pp. 70–71, and ''Storing Perishable Foods in the Home,'' Home and Garden Bulletin no. 78, U.S. Department of Agriculture.

Guide to selection and storage of fruits

Fruit	SELECTION CRITERIA		Storage
	Desirable qualities	Characteristics to avoid	
Apples	Firm; crisp; good color for the variety of apple	Overripe; soft and mealy; bruises	Store mellow apples uncovered in the refrigerator; unripe or hard apples are best held at cool room temperature (60°–70°F) until ready to eat; use ripe apples within a month
Apricots	Uniform, golden color; plump; juicy; barely soft	Soft or mushy; hard; pale yellow or green color	Apricots may be ripe when purchased; if not, store at room temperature until flesh begins to soften, then refrigerate and use within 3–5 days
Avocados	Firm if to be used later, slightly soft for immediate use	Dark patches; cracked surfaces	Allow avocados to ripen at room temperature, then refrigerate; use within 3–5 days
Bananas	Firm; bright color; free from bruises	Bruises; discolored skin	Allow bananas to ripen at room temperature, then refrigerate; the skin on bananas will darken but the flesh will remain flavorful and firm; use within 3–5 days
Blueberries	Dark blue with silver bloom; plump; firm; uniform size	Soft, spoiled berries; stems and leaves	Store covered in refrigerator to prevent moisture loss; do not wash or stem before storing; use within 2–3 days
Cherries	Dark color in sweet cherries, bright red in pie cherries; glossy; plump	Shriveling; dull appearance; soft, leaking fruit; mold	Store covered in refrigerator to prevent moisture loss; do not wash or stem before storing; use within 2–3 days
Cranberries	Plump and firm; lustrous; red color	Soft and spongy; leaking	Store covered in refrigerator; use within 1 week

	SELECTION CRITERIA		
Fruit	Desirable qualities	Characteristics to avoid	Storage
Grapefruit	Firm; well shaped; heavy for size; thin skin indicates juiciness	Soft and discolored areas; mold	Stored best at a cool room temperature (60°–70°F); use within 2 weeks; may also be stored uncovered in the refrigerator
Grapes	Plump; yellowish cast for white or green grapes, red color predominating for red grapes; stems green and pliable	Soft; wrinkled; bleached area around stem; leaking	Grapes are ready to use when purchased; refrigerate and use within 3–5 days
Lemons	Rich yellow color (pale or greenish yellow for higher acid content); firm; heavy	Hard or shriveling; soft spots; mold; dark yellow	Stored best at a cool room temperature (60°–70°F); use within 2 weeks; may also be stored uncovered in the refrigerator
Limes	Glossy skin; heavy	Dry skin; decay	Stored best at cool room temperature (60°–70°F); use within 2 weeks; may also be stored uncovered in the refrigerator
Melons			
Cantaloupes	Smooth area where stem grew; bold netting; yellowish cast to the skin	Soft rind; bruises	For all melons: keep at room temperature until ripe, then refrigerate; when storing, cut melon, cover, and refrigerate
Casaba	Yellow rind; slight softening at blossom end	Decayed spots	
Crenshaw	Deep golden rind; very slight softening of rind; good aroma	Decayed spots	
Honeydew	Faint odor; yellow to creamy rind; slight softening at blossom end	Greenish-white rind; hard and smooth skin	

Guide to selection and storage of fruits (continued)

Fruit	SELECTION CRITERIA		Storage
	Desirable qualities	Characteristics to avoid	
Persian	Same as cantaloupe	Same as cantaloupe	
Watermelons	Slightly dull rind; creamy color on the underside	Cracks; dull rind	
Nectarines	Slight softening; rich color; plump	Hard or shriveled; soft	Nectarines may be ripe when purchased; if not, store at room temperature until flesh begins to soften; then refrigerate and use within 3–5 days
Oranges	Firm and heavy; bright, fresh skin, either orange or green tint	Light weight; dull skin; mold	Stored best at a cool room temperature (60–70°F); use within 2 weeks; may also be stored uncovered in the refrigerator
Peaches	Slightly soft; yellow color between the red areas	Very firm, hard; green ground color; very soft; decay	Peaches may be ripe when purchased; if not, store at room temperature until flesh begins to soften; then refrigerate and use within 3–5 days
Pears	Firm, but beginning to soften; good color for variety (Bartlett, yellow; Anjou or Cornice, light green to yellow green; Bosc, greenish yellow with skin russeting; Winter Nellis, medium to light green)	Weakening around the stem; shriveled; spots	Allow to ripen at room temperature, then refrigerate; use within 3–5 days

Fruit	Desirable qualities	Characteristics to avoid	Storage
Pineapples	Good pineapple odor; green to yellow color; spike leaves easily removed; heavy for size	Bruises; poor odor; sunken or slightly pointed pips	Pineapples will not ripen further after purchase and there will not be any increase in sugars during storage; use pineapple as soon as possible, as holding results in deterioration; once cut, pineapple may be stored in a tightly covered container 2–3 days
Plums	Good color for variety; fairly firm	Hard or shriveled; poor color; leaking	Plums are generally ripe when sold; refrigerate and use within 3–5 days
Raspberries	Good color for kind; plump; clean; no caps	Mold; leaking	Store covered in refrigerator to prevent moisture loss; do not wash or stem before storing; use within 2–3 days
Strawberries	Good red color; lustrous; clean; cap stem attached	Mold; leaking; large seeds	Store covered in refrigerator to prevent moisture loss; do not wash or stem before storing; use within 2–3 days

Chart adapted from: Margaret McWilliams, *Food Fundamentals,* 2nd ed. (New York: Wiley, 1974), pp. 108–10, and ''Storing Perishable Foods in the Home,'' Home and Garden Bulletin no. 78, U.S. Department of Agriculture.

How to reduce nutrient loss

Type of loss	Cause	Nutrients lost	To reduce losses
SOLUTION	Nutrients dissolve into water or watery solutions during preparation and cooking	Minerals, vitamin C, and B-complex vitamins	Avoid soaking foods unless necessary; use soaking liquid in cooking
			Use cooking methods that require the least amount of water, such as steaming, stir frying, waterless or pressure cooking
			Shorten cooking time: 1. Cook vegetables only to crisp—not mushy 2. Cover pan so that heat is retained 3. Decrease cooking time by starting foods on a hot pan or hot cooking element, or in boiling water
			Use cooking liquids and meat drippings for soups, gravies, sauces; remember to discard fat from meat drippings
DESTRUCTION	Heat	Thiamin, vitamin C, pyridoxine, folic acid, vitamin B_{12}, riboflavin	Reduce cooking time of vegetables as described above
			For meats: 1. Cook braised and stewed meats only long enough to become tender 2. Oven roast only to rare or medium stage 3. Pressure-cook
DESTRUCTION	Light	Folic acid, riboflavin, pyridoxine, vitamin B_{12}, vitamin E, vitamin A, vitamin K	Do not allow milk to stand in light; keep in cartons or brown glass bottles
			Do not add baking soda to green vegetables during cooking

Type of loss	Cause	Nutrients lost	To reduce losses
DESTRUCTION	Oxidation	Vitamin A, carotene, vitamin C, vitamin E, vitamin K, thiamin, pyridoxine, biotin, folic acid	Leave foods in as big pieces as possible to minimize exposure for oxidation
			Do not chop or slice foods too far in advance of serving or cooking
			Inactivate quickly enzymes that cause oxidation by adding foods (especially vegetables) to heat, i.e., to boiling water, to hot cooking element or pan
			Use acids to inactivate enzymes, especially in salads (e.g., lemon juice, vinegar)
			Refrigerate or freeze foods in order to slow enzyme activity
			Keep produce fresh and crisp by storing properly

Note: *Phytate* (*phylic acid*), which is found in whole grains, has the capacity to bind the minerals calcium, zinc, and iron. Minimize this binding effect by having whole-grain breads that are leavened with yeast. The conditions required for leavening activate the enzyme phytase, which helps break down the phylic acid, making it unable to bind the minerals.

The minerals calcium and iron are also bound to a substance called *oxalic acid,* which is found in spinach, chard, sorrel, parsley, beet greens, rhubarb, and chocolate. Therefore don't count on these foods to supply your total source of calcium and iron.

Recommended daily dietary allowances
DESIGNED FOR THE MAINTENANCE OF GOOD NUTRITION OF PRACTICALLY ALL HEALTHY PEOPLE IN THE UNITED STATES.[a]

	Age	Weight		Height		Protein	FAT-SOLUBLE VITAMINS Vitamin A	Vitamin D	Vitamin E
	(years)	(kg)	(lbs)	(cm)	(in)	(g)	(μg R.E.)[b]	(μc)[c]	(mg $\propto$ T.E.)[d]
INFANTS	0.0–0.5	6	13	60	24	kg x 2.2	420	10.0	3
	0.5–1.0	9	20	71	28	kg x 2.0	400	10.0	4
CHILDREN	1–3	13	29	90	35	23	400	10.0	5
	4–6	20	44	112	44	30	500	10.0	6
	7–10	28	62	132	52	34	700	10.0	7
MALES	11–14	45	99	157	62	45	1000	10.0	8
	15–18	66	145	176	69	56	1000	10.0	10
	19–22	70	154	177	70	56	1000	7.5	10
	23–50	70	154	178	70	56	1000	5.0	10
	51+	70	154	178	70	56	1000	5.0	10
FEMALES	11–14	46	101	157	62	46	800	10.0	8
	15–18	55	120	163	64	46	800	10.0	8
	19–22	55	120	163	64	44	800	7.5	8
	23–50	55	120	163	64	44	800	5.0	8
	51+	55	120	163	64	44	800	5.0	8
PREGNANT						+30	+200	+5.0	+2
LACTATING						+20	+400	+5.0	+3

[a]The allowances are intended to provide for individual variations among most normal persons as they live in the United States under usual environmental stresses. Diets should be based on a variety of common foods in order to provide other nutrients for which human requirements have been less well defined.

[b]Retinol equivalents. 1 retinol equivalent = 1μg retinol or 6μg β-carotene.

[c]As cholecalciferol. 10μg cholecalciferol = 400 I.U. vitamin D

[d]$\propto$ tocopherol equivalent. 1 mg d-$\propto$ tocopherol = 1 $\propto$ T.E.

[e]1 N.E. (niacin equivalent) is equal to 1 mg of niacin or 60 mg of dietary tryptophan.

Vitamin C (mg)	Thiamin-B$_1$ (mg)	Riboflavin-B$_2$ (mg)	Niacin (mg N.E.)[e]	Vitamin B$_6$ (mg)	Folacin (µg)	Vitamin B$_{12}$ (µg)	Calcium (mg)	Phosphorus (mg)	Magnesium (mg)	Iron (mg)	Zinc (mg)	Iodine (µg)
35	0.3	0.4	6	0.3	30	0.5[f]	360	240	50	10	3	40
35	0.5	0.6	8	0.6	45	1.5	540	360	70	15	5	50
45	0.7	0.8	9	0.9	100	2.0	800	800	150	15	10	70
45	0.9	1.0	11	1.3	200	2.5	800	800	200	10	10	90
45	1.2	1.4	16	1.6	300	3.0	800	800	250	10	10	120
50	1.4	1.6	18	1.8	400	3.0	1200	1200	350	18	15	150
60	1.4	1.7	18	2.0	400	3.0	1200	1200	400	18	15	150
60	1.5	1.7	19	2.2	400	3.0	800	800	350	10	15	150
60	1.4	1.6	18	2.2	400	3.0	800	800	350	10	15	150
60	1.2	1.4	16	2.2	400	3.0	800	800	350	10	15	150
50	1.1	1.3	15	1.8	400	3.0	1200	1200	300	18	15	150
60	1.1	1.3	14	2.0	400	3.0	1200	1200	300	18	15	150
60	1.1	1.3	14	2.0	400	3.0	800	800	300	18	15	150
60	1.0	1.2	13	2.0	400	3.0	800	800	300	18	15	150
60	1.0	1.2	13	2.0	400	3.0	800	800	300	10	15	150
+20	+0.4	+0.3	+2	+0.6	+400	+1.0	+400	+400	+150	[g]	+5	+25
+40	+0.5	+0.5	+5	+0.5	+100	+1.0	+400	+400	+150	[g]	+10	+50

[f] The RDA for vitamin B$_{12}$ in infants is based on average concentration of the vitamin in human milk. The allowances after weaning are based on energy intake (as recommended by the American Academy of Pediatrics) and consideration of other factors such as intestinal absorption.

[g] The increased requirement during pregnancy cannot be met by the iron content of habitual American diets nor by the existing iron stores of many women; therefore the use of 30 to 60 mg of supplemental iron is recommended. Iron needs during lactation are not substantially different from those of nonpregnant women, but continued supplementation of the mother for two to three months after parturition is advisable in order to replenish stores depleted by pregnancy.

From: Recommended Daily Dietary Allowances, Revised 1979. Food and Nutrition Board, National Academy of Sciences–National Research Council, Washington, D.C.

A few of these simple changes in your habits will unquestionably increase the amount of vitamins and minerals you eat. Before reaching for a vitamin supplement, rethink the way you select, store, and prepare food.

Part 8

Putting it all together

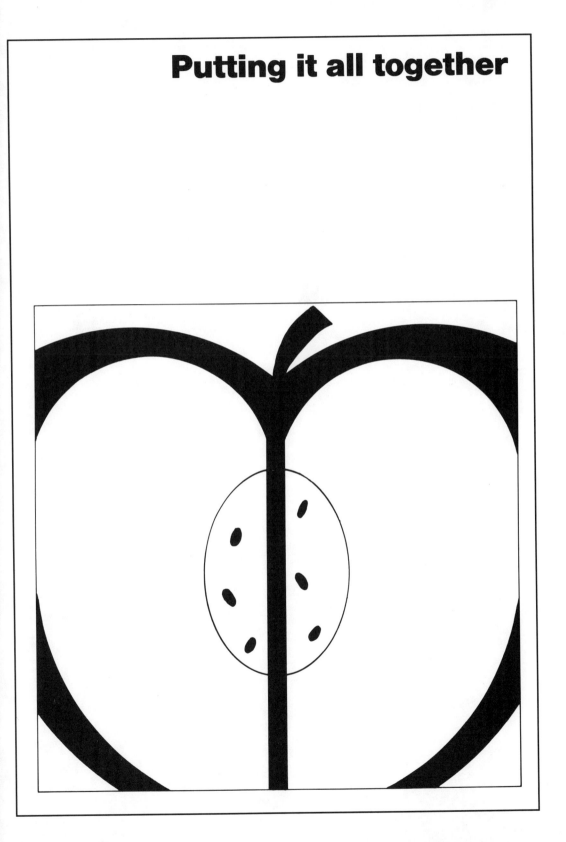

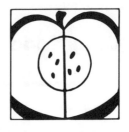

Having considered so many different aspects of your eating habits, you may feel somewhat confused about putting it all together to achieve a balanced diet. Well, don't worry. Good, healthful eating is really quite simple. In general, keep the following points in mind when choosing your foods:

- Eat a variety of *minimally processed* foods.

- Keep "empty" sugar calories to a minimum.

- Watch out for fats. Limit total fat, saturated fats, and cholesterol.

- Eat meatless meals several times each week.

- Include whole-grain breads and cereals in your diet.

- Eat fruits and vegetables daily.

- Minimize the amount of highly refined, processed foods that you eat.

- Minimize the use of salt.

- Keep calories at a level that will maintain your ideal body weight.

☐ Basic food guide

Read through the "Daily Food Guide" on pages 150–53. This guide outlines the essentials of a balanced diet and is specific about the kinds of foods and number of servings required.

If you select foods from each group in the amounts suggested, you will have a total calorie count of 915 to 1,585 calories. Most people require more calories than this in order to maintain an ideal body weight. (See "A Few Guidelines for Meal Planning," page 161.) Therefore, when planning your menus, you may add extra servings to meet your caloric requirements.

If you are trying to lose weight, you will do well to stay close to the amounts outlined on the chart. If you wish to be more specific about the calories in foods you choose, see the "Calorie Chart," pages 29–44.

Daily food guide

Food group	Daily servings	Average serving size
Milk and milk products	2 servings	1 cup: skim milk, low-fat milk (1–2%), buttermilk—skim, low-fat yogurt—plain 1 oz cheese
Vegetables (low starch vegetables)	2 servings—include at least one serving of a dark green or deep yellow vegetable	½ cup: spinach, broccoli, turnip greens, carrots, green beans, eggplant, tomatoes, asparagus, cauliflower, zucchini, etc.
Fruits	2 servings—include at least one fruit high in vitamin C	Small apple ½ banana 2 dates 1 fig ½ cup grapefruit or orange juice ½ grapefruit ¼ cup grape juice ½ small mango ¼ cantaloupe 1 small nectarine 1 small orange 1 medium peach 2 medium plums 2 medium prunes ¼ cup prune juice 2 tablespoons raisins 1 medium tangerine
Breads, pastas, other grains, and starchy vegetables	4 servings	1 slice whole-grain bread ½ whole-wheat English muffin 1 tortilla (6″) 3 tbsp dried bread crumbs 1 oz ready-to-eat cereal ½ cup: cooked cereal, cornmeal grits, pasta, rice, winter squash, mashed potato ⅓ cup corn ¼ cup sweet potato 2 squares graham crackers 3 rye wafers 1 small white potato

Approximate calories per serving	Nutritional contributions	Comments
90–150	Leading source of calcium in the diet; also important for phosphorus, magnesium, high-quality protein, vitamins A and D (if fortified), B-complex vitamins	Select low-fat milk products to limit total fat, saturated fat, cholesterol, and calories; choose low-fat milk fortified with vitamins A and D—otherwise these vitamins are removed with the fat
25	Important sources of vitamin A (as carotene); vegetables also supply vitamin C, B-complex vitamins, minerals, and fiber	Select, store, and prepare vegetables carefully to retain vitamins and minerals (see pp. 135–37)
40–80	Fruits high in vitamin C include grapefruit, grapefruit juice, orange, orange juice, cantaloupe, mango, fresh strawberries; fruits also supply vitamin A (as carotene), folic acid, potassium, and fiber	Select, store, and prepare fruits carefully in order to retain vitamins and minerals (see pp. 138–41)
55–110	Whole grains are important for their complex carbohydrates, B vitamins, minerals, fiber, and some incomplete protein	Whole grains contain important nutrients missing in refined products; although enriched, refined flours are good sources of iron and B vitamins, the refining process removes fiber and micronutrients found in the original grain; have yeast-leavened whole-wheat bread in order to destroy phytates that bind iron and zinc

Daily food guide (continued)

Food group	Daily servings	Average serving size
Meat substitutes	4 servings	½ cup cooked beans, peas, lentils (legumes) 2 tbsp peanut butter (equals 1 meat serving and 2 fat servings) 1 egg (limit to 3 per week) ½ cup cottage cheese 1 oz cheese (also in milk group; limit to 4 oz per week) ⅔ piece tofu (⅔ of piece that is 2½″ × 2¾″ × 1″)
Meats	1 serving	3–4 oz: fish, poultry, lean beef, lean lamb, lean pork
Fats and oils	3 servings	1 tsp oil, margarine, mayonnaise 1 tbsp salad dressing 10 whole peanuts 6 small other nuts 1 tbsp seeds 1 tbsp peanut butter (and ½ meat serving)
Fluid	48–64 oz (1½–2 qts)	

Approximate calories per serving	Nutritional contributions	Comments
55–110	Beans, peas, and lentils are important sources of B vitamins (not B_{12}), protein (incomplete), calcium, iron, zinc, fiber, and complex carbohydrates	Legumes provide protein as well as complex carbohydrates and fiber
165–220	Lean meats provide high-quality protein, iron, zinc, and B vitamins	The fat in red meats contains cholesterol and saturated fat; limit animal fats by having more fish, poultry, and meat substitutes
40–80	Calories, essential fatty acids, vitamin A, vitamin D	Remember, fats are the richest source of calories; fats from vegetable sources contain no cholesterol; vegetable oils (other than coconut and palm oils) are rich in polyunsaturated fats
	Helps body to dissolve and digest food, to carry nutrients to and from the body, to give shape and size to muscle and other parts of the body, and to keep an even body temperature	Obtain fluid from water, milk, fruit juices, and other beverages

☐ Some sample menus

Browse through the sample menus on the following pages. These examples are included to help you incorporate foods from the basic groups into your daily meals.

The first three menus total approximately 1,200 calories each and can be used as a guide for weight reduction. (Remember, consult your physician before you start a weight control program.) The second group of menus shows meals with a caloric level of approximately 2,000 calories per day. These meals would serve to maintain body weight for a woman who weighs 135 pounds and is moderately active or a man who weighs 150 pounds and is sedentary. Use the guidelines on page 161 (under the heading "A Few Guidelines for Meal Planning") to calculate the number of calories you require to maintain your weight. Then, alter your daily menus accordingly, to meet your caloric needs.

These menus illustrate just a few alternatives for a well-balanced diet. You may choose very different meal patterns from those illustrated to better suit your food preferences and life-style. For example, you may prefer to eat a bigger breakfast with a light lunch and a light meal in the evening. Also, frequent small meals may make you feel better, but remember to keep them small.

1,200 calorie diet

MENU 1

	Food	Portion size	Number food-group servings
BREAKFAST	Stewed prunes	4 prunes	2 fruit
	Cooked oatmeal	¾ cup	1½ bread
	Skim milk	1 cup (8 oz)	1 milk
	Beverage*		
LUNCH	Lentil soup	1 cup	1 vegetable, 1 meat substitute
	Cottage cheese	½ cup low-fat	1 meat substitute
	Carrot sticks	1 carrot	1 vegetable
	Cucumber slices	½ small cucumber	½ vegetable
	Tomato wedges	½ tomato	½ vegetable
	Rye crackers	3 crackers	1 bread
	Fresh orange	1 small	1 fruit
	Beverage*		
DINNER	Grapefruit juice	4 oz	1 fruit
	Broiled salmon cooked with:	5 oz (cooked)	1½ meat
	Margarine	1 tsp	1 fat
	Brown rice	½ cup cooked	1 bread
	Cooked spinach	½ cup	1 vegetable
	Beverage*		
SNACK	Skim milk	1 cup	1 milk
	Graham cracker	1 square	1 bread

*Includes beverages without calories such as water (tap or bottled), club soda, teas (herb or regular), coffee (limit because of caffeine)

1,200 calorie diet (continued)

MENU 2

	Food	Portion size	Number food-group servings
BREAKFAST	Orange juice	½ cup (4 oz)	1 fruit
	Shredded wheat	1 large biscuit	1 bread
	Skim milk	1 cup (8 oz)	1 milk
	Beverage*		
LUNCH	Vegetable barley soup	1½ cups	1½ meat substitute 1½ vegetable
	Peanut butter sandwich:		
	Peanut butter	2 tbsp	2 fat, 1 meat substitute
	Whole-grain bread	2 slices	2 bread
	Cantaloupe	¼ small	1 fruit
	Beverage*		
DINNER	Mushroom omelet cooked with:	2 eggs	2 meat substitute
	Margarine	2 tsp	2 fat
	Whole-wheat roll	½ med	1 bread
	Green salad with lettuce, broccoli, carrots, bean sprouts	1½ cups	3 vegetable
	Italian dressing	1 tbsp	1 fat
	Yogurt with:	1 cup low-fat	1 milk
	Banana	1 small	2 fruit
	Beverage*		

*Includes beverages without calories such as water (tap or bottled), club soda, teas (herb or regular), coffee (limit because of caffeine)

MENU 3

	Food	Portion size	Number food-group servings
BREAKFAST	Yogurt with:	1 cup low-fat	1 milk
	Apple	½ small	½ fruit
	Raisins	1 tbsp	½ fruit
	Whole-wheat toast with:	1 slice	1 bread
	Margarine	1 tsp	1 fat
	Beverage*		
LUNCH	Tomato soup (made with skim milk)	1½ cup	1 vegetable, 1 milk
	Chicken sandwich:		
	Cooked chicken	2 oz (cooked)	½ meat
	Mayonnaise	2 tsp	2 fat
	Whole-wheat bread	2 slices	2 bread
	Cold asparagus salad	5 med spears	1 vegetable
	Tangerine	1 med	1 fruit
	Beverage*		
DINNER	Vegetable juice	4 oz	1 vegetable
	Lean roast beef	4 oz (cooked)	1 meat
	Baked potato	1 small	1 bread
	Broccoli	1 med stalk	1 vegetable
	Margarine for potato and broccoli	1 tsp	1 fat
	Fresh grapefruit	½ med	1 fruit
	Beverage*		

*Includes beverages without calories such as water (tap or bottled), club soda, teas (herb or regular), coffee (limit because of caffeine)

2,000 calorie diet

MENU 1

	Food	Portion size	Number food-group servings
BREAKFAST	Orange juice	8 oz	2 fruit
	Cooked oatmeal	¾ cup	1½ bread
	Raisins	2 tbsp	1 fruit
	Skim milk	1 cup	1 milk
	Whole-wheat English muffin with:	1 muffin	2 bread
	Margarine	1 tsp	1 fat
	Beverage*		
LUNCH	Cheese lasagna	1 serving	2 meat substitute, 2 bread, 1 vegetable
	Green salad with lettuce, broccoli, carrots, bean sprouts	1½ cups	3 vegetable
	Italian dressing	1 tbsp	1 fat
	Whole-wheat Italian bread	1 slice	1 bread
	Tangerine	1 med	1 fruit
	Beverage*		
DINNER	Broiled salmon cooked with:	6 oz	2 meat
	Margarine	2 tsp	2 fat
	Brown rice	1 cup	2 bread
	Cooked spinach	1½ cups	1 vegetable
	Whole-wheat dinner roll	1 med	2 bread
	Margarine for vegetable and roll	1 tsp	1 fat
	Sliced banana	1 med	2 fruit
	Beverage*		
SNACK	Plain yogurt	1 cup	1 milk
	Apple	1 small	1 fruit

*Includes beverages without calories such as water (tap or bottled), club soda, teas (herb or regular), coffee (limit because of caffeine)

MENU 2

	Food	Portion size	Number food-group servings
BREAKFAST	Grapefruit juice	½ cup	1 fruit
	Bran flakes with:	1 cup	2 bread
	Fresh strawberries	½ cup	1 fruit
	Skim milk	1 cup	1 milk
	Whole-wheat toast with:	2 slices	2 bread
	Margarine	1 tsp	1 fat
	Low-fat cottage cheese	½ cup	1 meat substitute
	Beverage*		
LUNCH	Vegetable barley soup	1 cup	1 meat substitute, 1 vegetable
	Peanut butter sandwich:		
	Peanut butter	2 tbsp	2 fat, 1 meat substitute
	Whole-grain bread	2 slices	2 bread
	Dried figs	2	2 fruit
	Beverage*		
DINNER	Tomato juice	½ cup	1 vegetable
	Mushroom omelet cooked with:	2 eggs	2 meat substitute
	Margarine	2 tsp	2 fat
	Baked potato	1 med	2 bread
	Whole-wheat roll	1 med	2 bread
	Margarine for potato and roll	1 tsp	1 fat
	Green salad with lettuce, broccoli, carrots, bean sprouts	1½ cups	3 vegetables
	Italian dressing	1 tbsp	1 fat
	Yogurt with:	1 cup low-fat	1 milk
	Banana	1 small	2 fruit
	Beverage*		
SNACK	Dry roasted soynuts	½ cup	1 meat substitute

*Includes beverages without calories such as water (tap or bottled), club soda, teas (herb or regular), coffee (limit because of caffeine)

2,000 calorie diet (continued)

MENU 3

	Food	Portion size	Number food-group servings
BREAKFAST	Yogurt with:	1 cup low-fat	1 milk
	Apple	1 small	1 fruit
	Raisins	2 tbsp	1 fruit
	Wheat germ	¼ cup	1 bread
	Homemade bran muffin with:	1 med	2 bread
	Margarine	2 tsp	2 fat
	Beverage*		
LUNCH	Tomato soup (made with skim milk)	1½ cup	1 vegetable, 1 milk
	Chicken sandwich:		
	Cooked chicken	2 oz	½ meat
	Mayonnaise	1 tbsp	3 fat
	Whole-wheat bread	2 slices	2 bread
	Cold asparagus salad with:	5 med spears	1 vegetable
	Oil and vinegar	1 tbsp	1 fat
	Pear	1 small	1 fruit
	Beverage*		
DINNER	Vegetable juice cocktail	4 oz	1 vegetable
	Lean roast beef	4 oz (cooked)	1 meat
	Corn	⅔ cup	2 bread
	Broccoli	2 med stalks	2 vegetables
	Whole-wheat dinner roll	1 med	2 bread
	Margarine for vegetables and roll	2 tsp	2 fat
	Fresh grapefruit	½ med	1 fruit
	Beverage*		
SNACK	Grape juice	¾ cup (6 oz)	3 fruit
	Graham crackers	4 squares	2 bread

*Includes beverages without calories such as water (tap or bottled), club soda, teas (herb or regular), coffee (limit because of caffeine)

☐ Snacks

If you enjoy snacks, keep in mind that they are still part of the foods providing calories and nutrients for the day. This can be, and often is, a dangerous time for excess, empty-calorie foods. Many snack foods are also "junk foods," so called because they are often the highly refined, fatty, sugary, salty foods. This needn't be the case, however, for snacks can be as delicious and fun as they are nourishing.

Consider some alternatives to the commonly eaten snacks.

SNACK ALTERNATIVES

INSTEAD OF	HAVE	NUTRITIONAL BENEFITS
Doughnuts, Danish, a sweet roll	Homemade bran muffin, whole-wheat English muffin, or whole-wheat roll	Less sugar, more fiber, more trace minerals
Regular roasted, salted nuts	Dry roasted, unsalted soynuts	Fewer calories (225 fewer calories per ½ cup), less fat, less salt
Fruit-flavored, commercial yogurt	Plain yogurt with fresh fruit	Less sugar, more vitamins and minerals, more fiber, fewer calories
Colas and other sodas	Club soda with a twist of lemon or lime	Essentially no calories, no sugar, no food coloring, no caffeine
Chocolate bar	Carob-coated raisins	Less fat, more vitamins and minerals

☐ Getting started with meal planning

Lists, tables, and guidelines help set the stage for establishing new eating habits, but for them to become a reality, you need to go a step further. You are now ready to plan your new eating habits and to try them out. Find out which changes work well for you so that they can become a part of your daily routine. It is time to discard those habits that were working against you and to establish those that work for you.

A FEW GUIDELINES FOR MEAL PLANNING

- Review your "Personal Action Plans" for calories, carbohydrates, fat, protein, sodium, and vitamins and minerals. These plans clearly outline which changes in your present eating habits will improve your diet.

- Establish your caloric level by using the following formula. To *maintain* your body weight, calculate 15 calories for each pound that you weigh. This is the average for a moderately active person. For example, if you are moderately active and weigh 150 pounds, you would require approximately 2,250 calories per day to maintain this weight (15 calories/pound x 150 = 2,250 calories). If you are sedentary or get very little exercise, multiply your weight by 13. In this case the 150-pound person would require only 1,950 calories (13 calories/pound x 150 pounds = 1,950 calories) for weight maintenance. To *lose* weight, a deficit of 3,500 calories per pound per week is required. Subtract 500 calories per day to lose a pound a week or 1,000 calories per day to lose 2 pounds per week.

- Plan your meals ahead of time. What foods are you going to have? How many meals will you have? Will snacks be included? A little planning will make it easy to get started with your new eating habits. A good way to plan ahead is to outline a weekly food plan. By making decisions in advance you are setting yourself up to succeed in making changes. This type of planning is a good habit to acquire not only for your nutrition budget but also for your food budget.

Shopping is easier and more efficient when you have thought ahead. Remember to use your "Personal Action Plans," "Daily Food Guide," and "Calorie Chart" in making your food choices.

☐ Thoughts about food shopping

Careful selection of foods is an important step to eating well. We have available to us such a variety of foods that thought must go into choosing what we buy. Even items within the same food category can vary a great deal depending upon the quality, degree of processing, and additives in the food.

Keep these points in mind when buying food:

- Select fresh fruits and vegetables that are high in quality. (See guidelines, pages 135–41.)

- Select fresh fish, poultry, and red meats that have good color and little fat.

- When buying processed foods, read labels to:
  Minimize sugar.
  Minimize fat.
  Minimize salt.
  Avoid excessive food additives.

☐ Beware of additives

There is a great deal of controversy—and many unanswered questions—concerning food additives. Many are useful preservatives or nutrient and flavor enhancers, while others seem to be unnecessary and even potentially harmful.

It is best to minimize food additives, especially those that are of questionable safety. Check the chart on the following pages.

Keep in mind, however, that if you buy products without preservatives special care must be taken in storing the food. This is especially true for items such as whole grains and polyunsaturated oils. These foods can easily become rancid, forming harmful by-products. Store them in cool areas in airtight containers. It is probably wise to make certain that oils have some preservative—such as vitamin E or alpha tocopherol, which is a good antioxidant. It should be in the oil naturally, but the process of extraction may destroy the natural vitamin E.

The following are actual package labels illustrating variations in food additives. Although they are both crackers, the ingredients are vastly different.

Cracker #1	Cracker #2
Ingredients: Whole-grain wheat and rye flour, wheat and barley flour, yeast, and salt.	Ingredients: Enriched wheat flour, hydrolyzed corn cereal solids, sugar, salt, whey, natural flavor, monosodium glutamate (MSG), egg whites, dextrose, cornstarch, sodium bicarbonate, onion powder, sodium acid pyrophosphate, chicken broth, hydrolyzed vegetable protein, lecithin, malted barley, flour, spice extractives and spices, calcium carbonate, turmeric oleoresin (color), yeast, sodium bisulfate, and annatto extract (color).

Both products are from the cracker section in a supermarket, but what a difference between them! Cracker #1 is primarily whole grain with very little in the way of additives. Cracker #2 is a highly processed food with refined flour, several refined sugars (listed as sugar and dextrose), and loaded with additives, some of which (such as MSG and colorings) are better avoided.

These two labels represent only one example of the wide range in choice available to us when selecting our foods. It's all there—the many delicious, healthful foods along with those that may not be so good for us.

The choice is up to you.

Safety of common food additives

AVOID

Artificial Colorings: Most are synthetic chemicals not found in nature. Some are safer than others, but names of colorings are not listed on label. Used mostly in foods of low nutritional value, usually indicating that fruit or natural ingredient omitted.

ADDITIVE	USE	COMMENT
Blue No. 1	In beverages, candy, baked goods	Very poorly tested
Blue No. 2	Pet food, beverages, candy	Very poorly tested
Citrus red No. 2	Skin of some Florida oranges	May cause cancer; does not seep through into pulp
Green No. 3	Candy, beverages	Needs better testing
Orange B	Hot dogs	Causes cancer in animals
Red No. 3	Cherries in fruit cocktail, candy, baked goods	May cause cancer
Red No. 40	Soda, candy, gelatin desserts, pastry, pet food, sausage	Causes cancer in mice; widely used
Yellow No. 5	Gelatin dessert, candy, pet food, baked goods	Poorly tested; might cause cancer; some people allergic to it; widely used
Brominated vegetable oil (BVO)	Emulsifier, clouding agent for citrus-flavored soft drinks	Residue found in body fat; safer substitutes available
Butylated hydroxytoluene (BHT)	Antioxidant; cereals, chewing gum, potato chips, oils, etc.	May cause cancer; stored in body fat; can cause allergic reaction; safer alternatives
Caffeine	Stimulant, naturally in coffee, tea, cocoa; added to soft drinks	Causes sleeplessness; may cause miscarriages or birth defects
Quinine	Flavoring; tonic water, quinine water, bitter lemon	Poorly tested; some possibility that it may cause birth defects
Saccharin	Noncaloric sweetener; "diet" products	Causes cancer in animals
Sodium nitrite, sodium nitrate	Preservative, coloring, flavoring; bacon, ham, frankfurters, luncheon meats, smoked fish, corned beef	Prevents growth of botulism bacteria, but can lead to formation of small amounts of cancer-causing nitrosamines, particularly in fried bacon

CAUTION

ADDITIVE	USE	COMMENT
Artificial coloring: Yellow No. 6	Beverages, sausage, baked goods, candy, gelatin	Appears safe, but can cause allergic reactions
Artificial flavoring	Soda, candy, breakfast cereals, gelatin desserts, etc.	Hundreds of chemicals used to mimic natural flavors, almost exclusively in "junk" foods; indicates "real thing" is left out; may cause hyperactivity in some children
Butylated hydroxyanisole (BHA)	Antioxidant; cereals, chewing gum, potato chips, oils	Appears safer than BHT but needs better testing; safer substitutes available
Heptyl paraben	Preservative, beer	Probably safe, has not been tested in presence of alcohol
Monosodium glutamate (MSG)	Flavor enhancer; soup, seafood, poultry, cheese, sauces, stews, etc.	Damages brain cells in infant mice; causes "Chinese restaurant syndrome" (headache and burning or tightness in head, neck, arms) in some sensitive adults
Phosphoric acid; phosphates	Acidifier, chelating agent, buffer, emulsifier, nutrient, discoloration inhibitor; baked goods, cheese, powdered foods, cured meat, soda, breakfast cereals, dried potatoes	Useful chemicals that are not toxic, but their widespread use creates dietary imbalance that may cause osteoporosis
Propyl gallate	Antioxidant; oil, meat products, potato sticks, chicken soup base, chewing gum	Not adequately tested; use is frequently unnecessary
Sulfur dioxide, sodium bisulfite	Preservative, bleach; sliced fruit, wine, grape juice, dried potatoes, dried fruit	Can destroy vitamin B_1, but otherwise safe

SAFE

Alginate, propylene, and glycol alginate	Thickening agent, foam stabilizer; ice cream, cheese, candy, yogurt	Derived from seaweed

Safety of common food additives
(continued)

ADDITIVE	USE	COMMENT
Alpha tocopherol	Antioxidant, nutrient; vegetable oil	Vitamin E
Ascorbic acid, erythorbic acid	Antioxidant, nutrient, color stabilizer; oily foods, cereals, soft drinks, cured meats	Ascorbic acid and its salt, sodium ascorbate, provide nutrient vitamin C; erythorbic acid has no value as vitamin; all help prevent formation of cancer-causing nitrosamines
Beta carotene	Coloring, nutrient; margarine, shortening, nondairy creamers, butter	Body converts it to vitamin A
Calcium (or sodium) propionate	Preservative; bread, rolls, pies, cakes	Prevents mold growth; calcium a nutrient
Calcium (or sodium) stearoyl lactylate	Dough conditioner, whipping agent; bread dough, cake fillings, artificial whipped cream, processed egg white	Sodium stearoyl fumerate, also safe, serves same function
Carrageenan	Thickening and whitening agent; ice cream, jelly, chocolate milk, infant formula	From "Irish moss" seaweed
Casein, sodium caseinate	Thickening and whitening agent; ice cream, ice milk, sherbet, coffee creamers	Nutritious, the principal protein in milk
Citric acid, sodium citrate	Acid, flavoring, chelating agent; ice cream, sherbet, fruit drink, candy, carbonated beverages, instant potatoes	Citric acid is abundant in citrus fruits and berries; an important metabolite
EDTA	Chelating agent; salad dressing, margarine, sandwich spreads, mayonnaise, processed fruits and vegetables, canned shellfish, soft drinks	Traps metallic impurities that would otherwise cause rancidity and discoloration
Ferrous gluconate	Coloring, nutrient; black olives	A source of nutrient iron
Fumaric acid	Tartness agent; powdered drinks, pudding, pie fillings, gelatin desserts	Safe, but to enhance solution in cold water, DSS added, a poorly tested, detergentlike additive

ADDITIVE	USE	COMMENT
Gelatin	Thickening, gelling agent; powdered dessert mix, yogurt, ice cream, cheese spread, beverages	From animal bones, hooves, and other parts; little nutritional value as protein
Glycerin (glycerol)	Maintains water content; marshmallow, candy, fudge, baked goods	Natural backbone of fat molecules; used as energy or to build complex molecules
Gums: locust bean, guar, furcelleran, Arabic, karaya, tragacanth, ghatti	Thickening, stabilizing agents; beverages, ice cream, frozen pudding, salad dressing, dough, cottage cheese, candy, drink mixes	Derived from bushes, trees or seaweed; poorly tested but probably safe
Hydrolyzed vegetable protein (HVP)	Flavor enhancer; instant soups, frankfurters, sauce mixers, beef stew	Vegetable (usually soybean) protein chemically broken down into constituent amino acids
Lactic acid	Acidity regulator; spanish olives, cheese, frozen desserts, carbonated beverages	Naturally occurring in almost all living organisms
Lactose	Sweetener; whipped topping mix, breakfast pastry	Slightly sweet carbohydrate from milk
Lecithin	Emulsifier, antioxidant; baked goods, margarine, chocolate, ice cream	Common in animals and plants; a source of the nutrient choline
Mannitol	Sweetener; chewing gum, low-calorie foods	Less sweet than sugar; because it is poorly absorbed by body, has only half the calories of sugar
Mono- and diglycerides	Emulsifiers; baked goods, margarine, candy, peanut butter	Safe, but used mostly in foods that are high in sugar or fat
Polysorbate 60, 65, and 80	Emulsifiers; baked goods, frozen desserts, imitation dairy products	Synthetic but appear to be safe
Sodium benzoate	Preservative; fruit juice, carbonated drinks, pickles, preserves	Used more than 70 years to prevent growth of microorganisms

Safety of common food additives
(continued)

ADDITIVE	USE	COMMENT
Sodium carboxymethylcellulose (CMC)	Thickening, stabilizing agent, prevents sugar from crystallizing; ice cream, beer, pie fillings, icings, diet foods, candy	Made by reacting cellulose with acetic acid (vinegar); studies indicate safety
Sorbic acid, potassium sorbate	Prevents mold, bacterial growth; cheese, syrup, jelly, cake, wine, dried fruits	From berries of mountain ash; sorbate may be safe substitute for sodium nitrite in bacon
Sorbitan monostearate	Emulsifier; cakes, candy, frozen pudding, icing	Keeps oil and water mixed
Sorbitol	Sweetener, thickening agent, moisturizer; dietetic drinks and foods, candy, shredded coconut, chewing gum	From fruits and berries, half as sweet as sugar; slowly absorbed, thus safe for diabetics
Starch, modified starch	Thickening agent; soup, gravy, baby foods	From flour, potatoes, corn; modified chemically to improve solution in cold water; used to make foods look thicker and richer
Vanillan, ethyl vanillan	Substitute for vanilla flavoring; ice cream, baked goods, beverages, chocolate, candy, gelatin desserts	Vanillan, synthetic version of main flavor in vanilla bean, is safe; ethyl vanillin has more authentic taste but needs more testing

SPECIAL CONSIDERATIONS

ADDITIVE	USE	COMMENT
Salt (sodium chloride)	Flavoring; most processed foods—soup, potato chips, crackers, cured meat, etc.	Large amounts of sodium may cause high blood pressure in susceptible people and increase risk of heart attack and stroke
Sugars: corn syrup, dextrose, glucose, invert sugar, sugar	Sweeteners; candy, soft drinks, cookies, syrups, toppings, sweetened cereals, and many other foods	Mostly in foods with low, if any, nutritional value; excess sugars may promote tooth decay and precipitate diabetes in susceptible persons; condensed source of calories

Eating is indeed one of the pleasures in life, and a good diet is both pleasurable and healthy. It is our wish that the Health Action Plan, *Nutrition,* has equipped you with a new awareness about potential problems in your dietary patterns, the knowledge to understand the importance of good nutrition, and the tools for making changes to improve eating habits. Enjoy eating well for life.

Sample record keeping forms

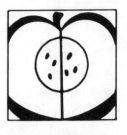

The sample form on the next page indicates how you might record your food intake for one week before taking the self-assessment tests in Parts 2 through 7. The sample on page 172 indicates how you might record all the statements to which you answered "no" in the self-assessment tests in Parts 2 through 7. These statements can serve as your personal goals for improving your eating habits.

SAMPLE FOOD RECORD

MEAL OR SNACK	FOOD	AMOUNT*
MORNING FOODS		
Breakfast	Orange juice	4 ounces
	Cheese Danish	1 average
	Coffee with:	1 cup
	Sugar	2 teaspoons
	Cream	2 tablespoons
Snack	Coffee with:	2 cups
	Sugar	4 teaspoons
	Cream	4 tablespoons
AFTERNOON FOODS		
Lunch	Cheeseburger including:	
	Hamburger	1 large
	American cheese	1 slice
	Bun	1 large
	French Fries	average serving
	Coke	1 large
Snack	Scotch	1 jigger
	Peanuts	1 handful
EVENING FOODS		
Dinner	Fried Chicken	1 breast
	White rice with:	1 cup
	Butter	1 pat
	Green peas	1/2 cup
	Tossed green salad with:	1 average
	Blue cheese dressing	2 tablespoons
	French Vanilla ice cream	2 scoops
	Coffee with:	1 cup
	Sugar	2 teaspoons
	Cream	2 tablespoons

*Estimate portion sizes as best you can in terms of ounces, cups, teaspoons, tablespoons, whenever possible. Otherwise, record as small, medium or large servings.

SAMPLE PERSONAL ACTION PLAN

FATS
- Have fish and poultry more frequently than red meats.
- Choose low-fat snacks (such as raw vegetables, fruits, whole-grain crackers, or plain yogurt) rather than nuts and chips.
- Have no more than one serving a week or none at all of high-fat luncheon meats (franks, bologna, salami, liverwurst, etc.).

PROTEIN
- Aim for a variety of vegetables in a meatless meal.
- Use legumes (beans, peanuts, and peas) of all kinds in cooking.
- Keep meat portions small (not more than an average of 3 to 4 ounces per day or 21 to 28 ounces a week.

Selected reading

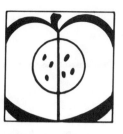

Bennet, I., and Simon, M. *The Prudent Diet.* New York: David White, Inc., 1975.

Brewster, Letitia, and Jacobson, Michael F. *The Changing American Diet.* Washington, D.C.: The Center for Science in the Public Interest, 1978.

Deutsch, Ronald M. *The New Nuts Among the Berries.* Palo Alto, California: Bull Publishing, 1977.

Fremes, Ruth, and Sabry, Zak. *NutriScore.* New York: Methuen/Two Continents Publications, 1976.

Glenn, Morton B. *But I Don't Eat That Much.* New York: E.P. Dutton & Co., Inc., 1974.

Gussow, Joan. *The Feeding Web.* Palo Alto, California: Bull Publishing, 1978.

Jordan, Henry A.; Levitz, Leonard S.; and Kimbrell, Gordon M. *Eating Is Okay.* New York: New American Library, Inc., 1976.

Konishe, Frank. *Exercise Equivalents of Foods.* London and Amsterdam: Feffer and Simons, Inc., 1976.

McGill, Marion, and Orrea, Pye. *The No-Nonsense Guide to Food and Nutrition.* New York: Butterick Publishing, 1978.

Recommended Dietary Allowances. Washington, D.C.: National Academy of Sciences, 1979.

Robertson, L.; Flinders, C.; and Godrey, B. *Laurel's Kitchen.* Petaluma, California: Nilgiri Press, 1976.

Dietary Goals for the United States. 2nd ed. Select Committee on Nutrition and Human Needs, United States Senate. Washington D.C.: United States Government Printing Office, 1977.

Index